stand tall like a mountain

For my cherubs Charlotte and Teddy, and for all children – may you feel empowered to stand tall like a mountain

An Hachette UK Company
www.hachette.co.uk

First published in Great Britain in 2019 by Aster, an imprint of
Octopus Publishing Group Ltd
Carmelite House
50 Victoria Embankment
London EC4Y 0DZ
www.octopusbooks.co.uk
www.octopusbooksusa.com

Text copyright © Suzy Reading 2019
Design and layout copyright © Octopus Publishing Group 2019

Distributed in the US by Hachette Book Group
1290 Avenue of the Americas
4th and 5th Floors, New York, NY 10104

Distributed in Canada by Canadian Manda Group
664 Annette Street,Toronto, Ontario, Canada M6S 2C8

ISBN 978-1-91202-395-0

A CIP catalogue record for this book is available from the British Library.

Printed and bound in China

10 9 8 7 6 5 4 3 2 1

Consultant publisher Kate Adams
Senior editor Pauline Bache
Copy editor Jane Birch
Art director Yasia Williams-Leedham
Illustrator Ella Mclean
Picture research manager Giulia Hetherington
Production manager Lisa Pinnell

stand tall like a mountain

Mindfulness & Self-Care for Children & Parents

Suzy Reading

aster

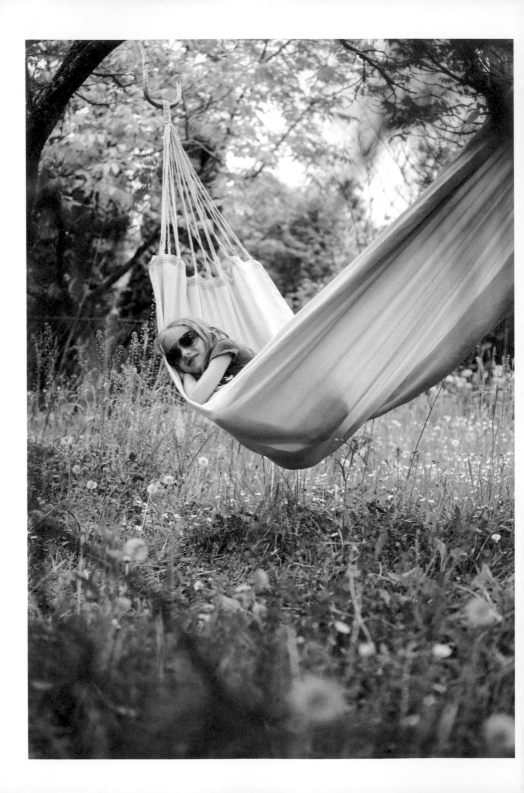

Contents

INTRODUCTION

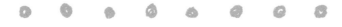

What makes for a buoyant mood? How do we stay connected with our calm abiding centre? What are those inner resources that help us weather life's inevitable curveballs? Over a decade ago a friend asked me how I maintained such an upbeat approach to life. Having grown up in a harsh eastern European climate, she assumed my sunny disposition was due to being raised on the beaches of Sydney, Australia. At the time, I didn't know the answer to her question, but as a psychologist, it really piqued my interest and I knew it was down to much more than just sunshine. In many ways, my friend was right – I'd had an idyllic childhood in a nourishing place which provided a solid bedrock. But life has a way of catching up with us. No one is immune to adversity. And in my struggle I came to know the answer to her question: I call it the ability to stand tall like a mountain.

With the passage of time, including the twists and turns of international relocation, and becoming a mother at the same time as losing my father, I came to understand the building blocks to resilience first-hand. Experiencing those challenges and finding myself in a state of energetic bankruptcy, I kept coming back to my friend's question, because I'd lost that upbeat way of being. I was too tired and too sad to be able to think straight and many of my regular life-giving activities had fallen away. But by consciously rebuilding my self-care toolkit and with one little "micro moment" of nourishment at a time, that ember of positivity was sparked again. In clawing my way back to vitality I learned the true transformative power of self-care – all those nurturing acts that top us up so that we can feel a sense of optimism, equanimity and resilience, the ability to stand tall like a mountain. This is also the name of a yoga pose described in this book – come into this shape and it will help you channel these skills in mind and body:

Optimism: hopefulness and confidence about the future, like the apex of the mountain, lifting skywards.

Equanimity: calmness and composure, especially in the face of adversity, like the body of the mountain, standing firm against life's challenges.

Resilience: toughness and capacity to bounce back after challenges, like the broad mountain base, anchoring us, helping us recover.

In navigating my grief, I reflected on the activities I engaged in as a child, so often led by my father: the clifftop walks, counting the types of birds we saw along the way, watching the rock fishermen reel in their catch or savouring a sunset together. It was in simple things such as hearing his joy at a favourite tune on the radio or his recounting a precious story of flying past some young jogger while running down a hill. In losing him, I reconnected with these practices and was reminded of how potent such things are for healing and for providing a protective buffer against future challenges. Now armed with the benefit of ten years' hindsight and supported by concrete findings from Positive Psychology on the foundations of well-being, I believe there are key skills and habits that contribute greatly to our mood, energy level, quality of mind and enjoyment of life, and these are skills and habits that we can all learn. I love that my self-care toolkit is a legacy of my father, and that I can share these same skills and habits with my children and see them blossom.

SELF-CARE IS THE SOLUTION

Self-care is a hot topic right now but the buzz concentrates primarily on adults. This book shifts the focus to preparing our children for the inevitable stresses of life, so they are best placed to care for themselves and cope when life gets tough. Stress is prevalent in the lives of our children – from jampacked schedules and the pressure to perform, to the advent of social media requiring management of an online life and the effects of screen time. Our children need their own self-care toolkit. It's about teaching them the tools of nourishment by engaging in self-care as a family, and showing them simple practices that they can turn to when they're on their own.

We teach our children how to brush their teeth, the importance of healthy eating and how to safely cross the road; this book aims to broaden their toolkit to include resilience-boosting skills and "emotional first aid", empowering them with methods to navigate difficult emotions and challenging life experiences. Rather than just hoping they'll absorb these skills by osmosis (that's if we parents are skilled in the art of self-care), this book will give you the tools to actively teach your kids how to engage in self-care, with practices specifically tailored for children to use independently and others to be enjoyed collectively. Many of the activities can be suitable from a very young age and so it's never too early to start introducing your children to ideas for self-care. Children are natural masters of curiosity and mindfulness, so the learning is not a one-way street. This book will encourage you to observe and seek opportunities to learn from your children too.

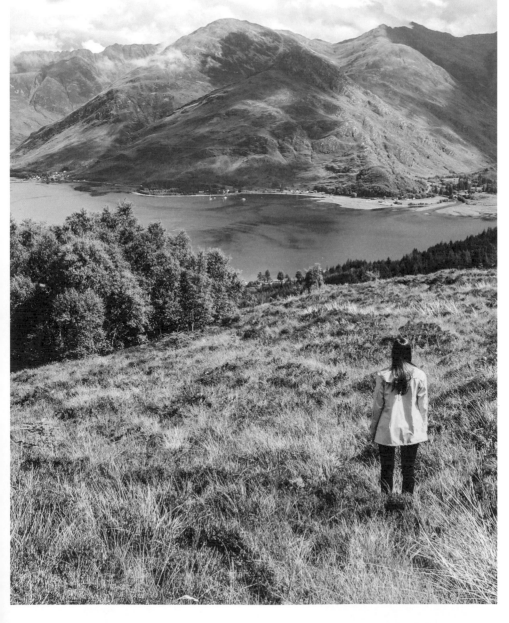

Self-care gives us the ability
to stand tall like a mountain

As a society, we are beginning to recognize the value and need for self-care and my practice as a psychologist now concentrates exclusively on empowering people with the tools of self-nourishment. A few years ago people were coming to me for help in creating their own healthy lifestyle changes. Many of these clients reflected that these skills and habits weren't demonstrated for them growing up. I now have more and more parents coming to me for help in developing a self-care toolkit that they can share with their children – and that's where the idea for this book was born. I sincerely hope you enjoy working through these concepts and practices with your cherubs and that the dividends ripple out for you all!

WHAT IS SELF-CARE?

While we have all heard of the term "self-care", it is still a bit fluffy and misunderstood. There is a good reason for this confusion and that's because as human beings we all need different things. What one person finds soothing or uplifting might not be a tonic for someone else and even our own needs change over time. Before we can effectively commit to engaging in self-care, we need a proper working definition and then we need a broad toolkit from which to draw.

To keep it as simple as possible, the mantra is "*self-care is health care*". It is nourishment for the head, the heart and the body. There is a second part of the definition that will help you get clear on what constitutes a true act of nourishment, and this is that self-care nurtures you in this moment, your "present self" if you like, but it also benefits the person you are becoming, your "future self". Adding this second part of the definition will stop your self-care from turning into an act of self-sabotage. One small bite of chocolate savoured may be self-care, but a whole bar of chocolate, which then scuppers the bedtime routine, will hardly have anyone feeling peaceful and nourished

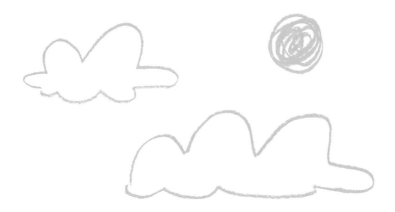

later on. When you are choosing an act of nourishment, just make sure your "present self" and your "future self" agree on it. It's worth acknowledging here that self-care is not always easy or comfortable. It's more than treats and pampering; sometimes the true act of self-care is the last thing you feel like doing.

The concept that helps bring self-care to life is the idea that we all have an "energy bank balance". Just as a car needs fuel to go, we need energy to power us through our day, our week, our month and our future. Self-care is any life-giving act that tops up your energy bank and the healthier your reserves, the better placed you are to cope with the daily challenges you face. If you're running on empty, you expose yourself to the risk of energetic bankruptcy. The car with an empty fuel tank is of use to no one and no one is immune. A regular self-care routine will boost your resilience and help you respond with greater resourcefulness to life as it happens, when the road is flat and smooth and, importantly, when we are facing that mountainous incline. It's no different for children.

WHY DO WE NEED SELF-CARE?

» **We need it to help us cope.** Stress, loss and change are inevitable parts of life, in childhood and adulthood. We all have difficult emotions and experiences to navigate, we all have a fallible human body and mind, and we all encounter loss in various forms – whether losing a loved one or getting used to saying goodbye to mum or dad at nursery. Self-care helps us cope in the moment.

» **We need it to help us recover.** Following on from challenges in our day, we need a self-care toolkit that is soothing and healing, helping us process and move through our feelings, thoughts, sensations and responses.

» **We need it to build a protective buffer from future challenges.** Proactively topping up your energy bank balance will keep you feeling more resilient and capable. In fact, when you are feeling vital and strong you interpret life differently to when you are depleted. Things that could potentially overwhelm you when you are fatigued might merely needle you when you are well nourished. You can interpret events as a minor irritation or an opportunity to grow when you are energetically topped up. We are all naturally more creative in our responses to problems when we have lovingly tended to our mental, emotional and physical health.

» **We need it to be our best self.** You're more likely to be the kind of person you aspire to be, achieving what you most desire, if you engage in self-care. Self-care is the means by which we become a better version of ourselves. We are all kinder, more patient, more productive people when we have nurtured ourselves head, heart and body. It truly is the ultimate win-win.

» **We need it to raise calm, compassionate and resilient children and for the collective health of the family unit.** Our children need to see us engaging in self-care to begin building their own toolkit. We need to be actively role-modelling these healthy behaviours for our kids and, better still, involving them in the practice of self-care, showing them why we need it and how to do it. It is not just of benefit to the individual; these practices have the potential to deepen bonds and boost the healthy functioning of the family unit itself. There is a positive upward spiral to be enjoyed which starts right here.

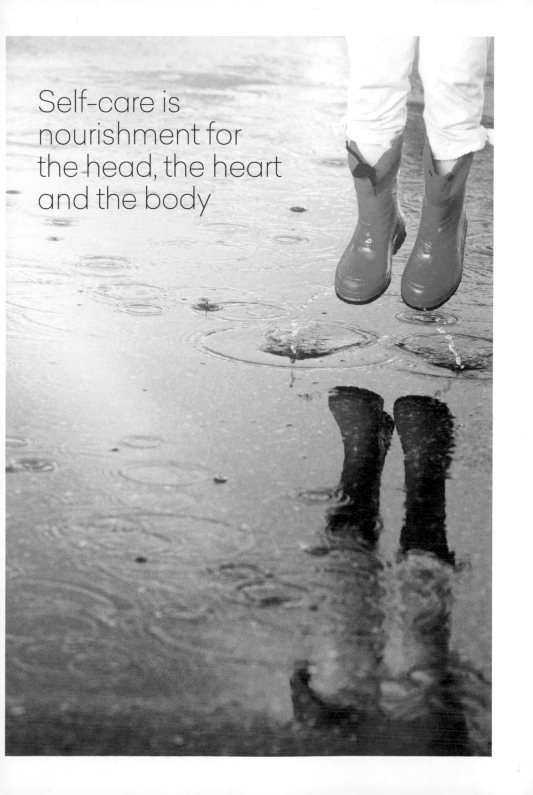

Self-care is
nourishment for
the head, the heart
and the body

HOW DO WE DO IT?

The most effective way to make self-care part of daily family life is to use a framework that will help you swiftly identify a form of self-care that is accessible and resonant, when you or your children need it the most. I created the Vitality Wheel framework for this purpose, and turning to it opens our eyes to the eight different ways, each reflected in a spoke of the Wheel, that we can nourish ourselves. They are not designed to be distinct and you'll see that one act of self-care could easily slot into a number of different spokes. The point of the Vitality Wheel is to get you connected with something to help you cope in an instant.

Think of the Vitality Wheel spokes as options, working with as many or as few as you and your children choose. You certainly don't have to engage in all spokes at the same time. Keep checking in with the Wheel and dipping into the corresponding chapters of the book as your child's and your family's interests naturally evolve. Many of these concepts and activities are common sense, and you will be doing plenty of the suggested activities already. There may, however, be some tools and ideas that are completely new to you and that's ok too. Some of these skills might feel tricky for us parents at first, and our children will naturally have a greater affinity with some tools, so again we can take delight in learning from them. In sharing with your children the tools that are new or challenging for you, you have an opportunity to demonstrate for them a "beginner's mind". Enjoy that you can explore developing these skills as beginners together. While I've certainly got the fitness side of things licked, I will put my hand up and freely admit that my cooking skills could do with some work. I love that my seven-year-old and I can be beginners together in the kitchen and in the process

I am teaching her much more than just cooking, I am teaching her how to develop a new skill with curiosity, relish and constructive inner dialogue, deepening our bonds and banking quality time together. We don't have to be good at all the things in the Vitality Wheel but, if we choose to, we all have opportunities to work on expanding our skill set and fine-tuning our abilities.

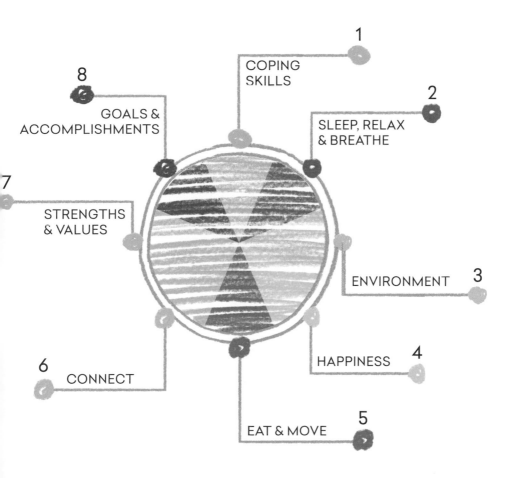

8 GOALS & ACCOMPLISHMENTS

1 COPING SKILLS

2 SLEEP, RELAX & BREATHE

7 STRENGTHS & VALUES

3 ENVIRONMENT

6 CONNECT

4 HAPPINESS

5 EAT & MOVE

"SELF-CARE IS HEALTH CARE" – INTUITIVE BUT NOT ALWAYS EASY!

Generally speaking, when we really need self-care, when we're feeling overwhelmed, fatigued or in the midst of anger, it can be very hard to think straight! So we do need to have our self-care toolkit written down. The best way is to annotate a copy of the Vitality Wheel so you can visually identify which form of nourishment grabs you, then you can take a closer look at one of the tools or strategies inspired by that spoke of the Vitality Wheel (see page 15).

We all know what we need to do to feel healthy but let's just be honest and recognize that self-care is not always easy and the healthy choice is not always the most alluring. Allow yourself to be human and then get organized to overcome the fact that willpower alone isn't enough to see us through. Creating a "Self-Care Journal" is a great way to overcome this challenge and can become a wellspring of inspiration and positivity.

YOUR SELF-CARE JOURNAL

I encourage parents to keep a journal for themselves and to work on one for each of their kids. For adults, your journal is about recording your goals and your choices, thereby boosting accountability and helping you to track progress, identify patterns and reflect on your accomplishments. It's also a place to record happy memories, write gratitude entries and collate images, letters, articles and quotes, just like you would on a vision board (see page 172) – you can get as creative as you like. For kids, it can be more of an arts and crafts approach, where entries are drawings or photos of the activities you've done together, and a place to create their own toolkits, for example, "What to do when I can't get to sleep". My daughter and I make an entry in her journal when we are discussing a challenge she has faced in her day and she often reflects on these entries at a later date, reinforcing her toolkit. We make entries about yoga poses, mindfulness techniques and gratitude practices and she can turn to her journal whenever she needs a boost of energy or a dollop of calm.

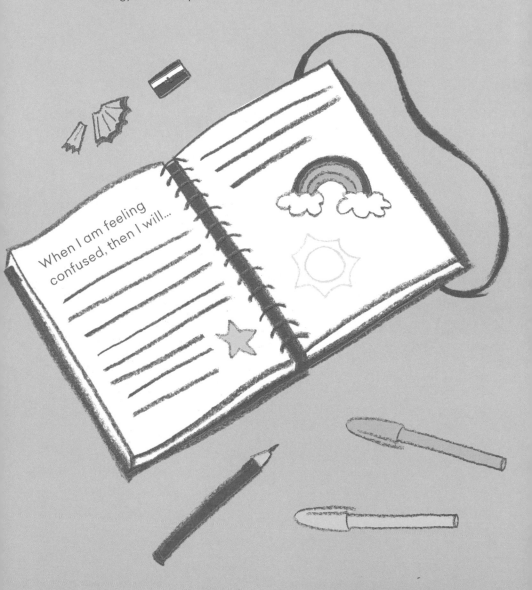

When I am feeling confused, then I will...

HOW TO USE THIS BOOK

This book is designed to be read by parents. There's a chapter on each spoke of the Vitality Wheel and each includes sections that you can read aloud and illustrations and practices you can share with your children. How you read it is totally up to you. If you want, you can read it cover to cover, or if you prefer, you can zip straight to the chapters which most resonate with you and your family. Sit down with your kids and engage in the activities together and refer to the text to learn about concepts that will help you guide your children through difficult emotions or the challenges they face.

The tips and tools in this book are informed by my studies and a decade of work as a psychologist and yoga teacher as well as my previous decade working as a personal trainer, both of which have been equally informative. I've learned that there truly is no separation between mental health and physical health and there are just different ways we can create change – either via the body, the mind or the breath. In every chapter you will find a range of activities from which to choose, some that use movement, some that harness the way we think and others involving either breathing, mindfulness or meditation. In my experience, the easiest way to change how you feel is to move your body. Movement is naturally appealing to children and is an easy way to cultivate the skill of mindfulness, so each chapter includes some yoga poses to try. Yoga can be a great starting point as you introduce the concept of self-care to your kids.

To help bring self-care to daily life, please use the ideas in the book to annotate your own Vitality Wheel. Simply jot down on a copy of the Wheel the activities that resonate most with you and your family and take some time to create your own self-care toolkit. Writing out your toolkit will help you all take swift, productive action whether you need a confidence boost or a feeling of peace. There are some sample toolkits to inspire you in common situations at the end of each chapter:

We need to get self-care on the radar for everyone. Talk about the self-care ideas you read in this book and have an open dialogue with your kids about your own toolkit. Share with your children why you are rolling out your yoga mat, let them join you and, yes, often that will mean they are climbing on your back. Show them the pose that you do before bed or the one that helps you feel brave. Or if you've never done yoga before, enjoy exploring the poses as beginners together. Talk about the kind of things you do when you're feeling anxious. Share with them the breathing techniques or coping strategies that work for you. When boredom descends or tempers flare on the weekend, refer to your annotated Vitality Wheel, and choose a nourishing act that you can all engage in together. The more we talk about self-care, the more salient our practices become and the more often we find ourselves engaging in these practices, with greater effect.

The aim of this book is to give you a wealth of options within fingertips' reach that take little time, energy or expense. With your encouragement, your children will grow up feeling that their self-care toolkit for emotional, mental and physical health is a normal part of life, just like brushing their teeth, and the benefits to them and the whole family can be profound. Enjoy exploring self-care with them and seeing those positive effects flow!

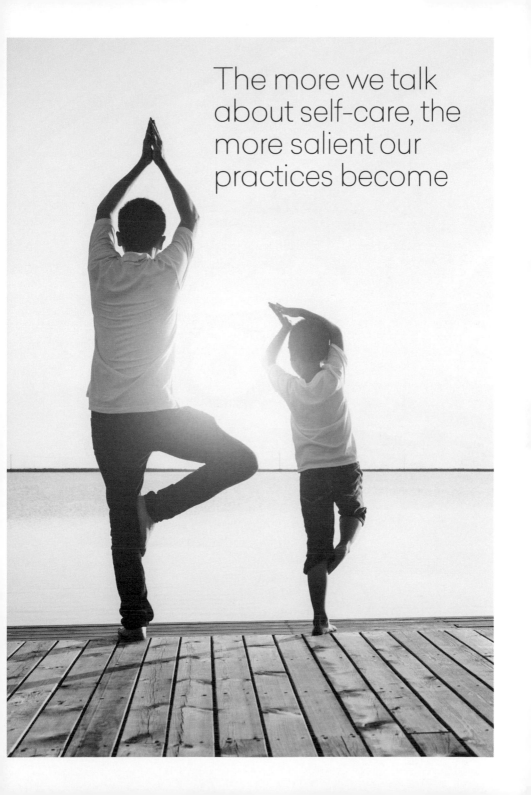

The more we talk about self-care, the more salient our practices become

ONE

· · · · · · · · ·

COPING SKILLS

Modern life is full and fast-paced for everyone. Our children face a different childhood landscape these days with new pressures and challenges to navigate – the overwhelming pressure to perform to "get ahead", breakfast club/after-school club, scheduling of extracurricular pursuits, screen and technology overload and, as they get older, managing an online life with social media. Just as there were public health campaigns in decades gone by on healthy eating and exercising, now we are seeing more messages about nurturing our mental and emotional health. This is with good reason because the prevalence of anxiety and depression is on the rise, touching not only adults but our children too. The good news is that there are plenty of habits and practices that can boost resilience and provide a protective buffer from stress. Adults and children alike are well served by having a broad set of coping tools from which to draw. This chapter introduces key concepts, such as mindfulness, emotional agility and growth mindset, in a way that will help you share them with your children. You will also learn specific practices and tools that will help you and your child navigate difficult emotions and challenging situations.

MINDFULNESS AS A COPING STRATEGY

If we want to live with a sense of peace and ease, mindfulness is an essential concept to embrace. It is a core coping skill in itself, helping us manage our thoughts and emotions, but also forming the foundation for many other self-care practices, such as savouring and gratitude, so we're going to dive into mindfulness first – what it means as a concept and practices that will help you and your family cultivate the ability to be mindful. Mindfulness is also fundamental to bringing self-care to life – without mindfulness it is impossible to know what you need! Mindfulness allows you to check in with your body and mind, to notice how you are feeling and then select the nourishing tool best suited to your needs. A family that is skilled in mindfulness will collectively cope better with stress, be able to respond to challenges with greater harmony and purpose and is able to truly enjoy the peak moments.

When you watch a child absorbed in play, you will see that they are already naturally skilled in aspects of mindfulness and we can learn a lot from this observation! As parents we can highlight this natural ability, showing them how to use this skill in other moments, talking them through the steps of how the same attention they give their play can help them nut out a problem, or move through a difficult emotion. Putting into words for them what mindfulness is and how they can do it will help them apply this skill throughout their day.

WHAT IS MINDFULNESS?

We recently made our first return visit to Australia after being away for four years – it's not only negative events that can throw us, even much desired events can trigger a cascade of big emotions to navigate! Without the skill of mindfulness I could have spent the entire two weeks lost in comparing UK and Sydney life, and grieving the future loss of my mother when she was sitting across the table from me! Mindfulness allowed me to notice and accept the maelstrom of feelings swirling about and to return my focus to the potential joy waiting to be experienced right in front of me. For my excited seven-year-old, the beginning of the trip was punctuated by queries about when we were going to do a myriad of things she remembered from her early childhood and mindfulness allowed her to be anchored in this one activity, safe in the knowledge that there would be time for other exciting things later. Towards the end of the trip, when collectively thoughts were turning to our departure, mindfulness helped us all stay in the moment, rather than squandering that time feeling sad that it was drawing to a close.

Mindfulness as a concept is being in touch with the present moment – what is happening in the environment around us and what is unfolding within us. Rather than being caught up in worry about the past or the future, mindfulness anchors us in the "now". It is noticing without judgment or resistance, our feelings, thoughts, sensations and memories, and the events happening around us. I think of mindfulness as a way of developing fresh eyes (and all the other sense organs), allowing us to connect with life as it unfolds, giving us space to choose how we respond rather than reacting blindly. Simply put, whatever you are doing right now, do that thing with your full attention. Aim to do that one thing and you are more likely to do it well and with less energetic drain. Multitasking is not all it's cracked up to be – notice how much juggling several things at once diminishes your productivity, increases your stress and frustration and depletes your energy bank.

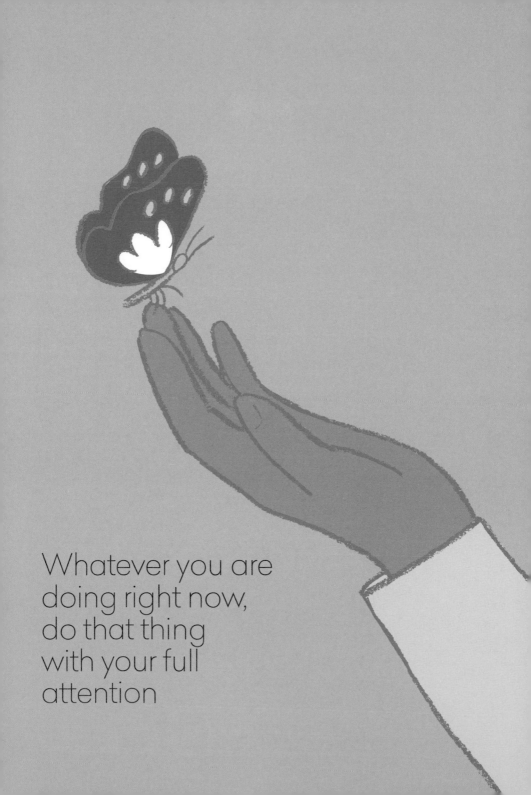

Whatever you are
doing right now,
do that thing
with your full
attention

At the heart of mindfulness lies the ability to be truly present, to notice and watch what is happening right now. It's experiencing life with real intention and wakefulness. At the same time, this focus needs to be coupled with a feeling of acceptance, allowing things to be as they are – the things we like, the things we're impartial to and the things we don't like. It is observing that this is the way things are right now. When we get lost in inner dialogue, judgment of our experience, or worry, we have lost that connection to what is happening in the moment. That's not to say that we have to be mindful in every moment. There is a time for getting lost in a daydream, for problem-solving – there is even a time for worry! Mindfulness puts us back in the driver's seat, allowing us to choose how we harness our minds.

Often it is our evaluation of what's happening right now that adds to our discomfort – thinking we mustn't feel like this, this shouldn't be happening, or it can't be like this... Mindfulness is seeing a thing the way it truly is, not resisting it or willing it away, because after all, it is happening, whether we like it or not. This is not to say we just sit back and let life wash over us. We still need to take action, but mindfulness creates the space to feel what we feel, to see a situation for what it is – the things we control and the things we can't control – and then empowers us with the opportunity to reflect on the best course of action. Mindfulness opens you up to truly experiencing life in its full glory – savouring precious moments, rather than frittering them away with divided attention, and helping you to weather the tougher times with less of a struggle.

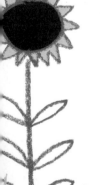

There is one more facet of mindfulness to share with your children. And this can be a bit of a light-bulb moment for them, and it was for me too! When we begin our journey with mindfulness we become super aware of our thoughts, emotions, memories and sensations. The key is to communicate to your child that they are not their thoughts, they *have* thoughts. They are not their emotions, they *feel* them. They are not their memories, they *experience* them. They are not their sensations, they *sense* them. This can be a liberating idea! Just as we experience the changing weather, we experience our thoughts, feelings, sensations and memories. You are far more magical than just a thought – you are the witness to all these passing states. It's what you do with your thoughts and emotions that matters. Language can help here too. Instead of labelling yourself "an angry person", reframe it as "I am feeling angry" which feels easier to deal with and only temporary. You can think a nasty thought but this does not then mean that you are a nasty person. Thoughts don't loom as large and prophetic – they were just passing thoughts, like passing showers or floating clouds. We'll explore this concept further in the mindfulness practices "Blue Sky Mind" (page 30) and your "Tending to your mind garden" (page 33).

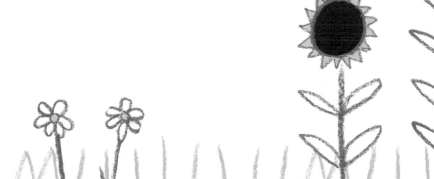

HOW DO WE DEVELOP THE SKILL OF MINDFULNESS?

A mindfulness practice is a constant process of bringing the mind back to "now", because the mind will wander and it will *always* be full of thoughts. Mindfulness is not about emptying the mind. The mind is designed to think just as the eyes are designed to see, so don't worry about trying to stop thoughts from coming. There are many different mindfulness practices to experiment with dotted through every chapter of this book and each of these will anchor the mind on different things such as the breath, thoughts, feelings, physical sensations, movement, eating, a phrase or a sound.

Starting even more simply than a formal practice, there are lots of children's games that are the perfect means to building your mindfulness muscles: jigsaws, Lego, the memory game, origami, colouring, Play-Doh and my favourite, Jenga, because it reminds my kids that making "mistakes" is part of life and not the end of the world. The key to making these activities a mindfulness practice is to give each one your full attention, with all your senses, and every time your mind wanders to judgment or other distractions, bring it back to the moment. Adults, please park your devices in another room, their mere presence will keep tugging at your attention.

You are not your thoughts, you *have* thoughts. You are not your emotions, you *feel* them

Practices to build mindfulness

Blue Sky Mind

Find a comfortable place to sit or lie down; this can be inside or outside, wherever you feel completely at ease. Close your eyes and just become aware. Feel your body, feel your breathing and notice your mind. Let all these thoughts, emotions, sensations and memories arise as they will. Don't resist them, don't engage with them, just notice them. Imagine in your mind's eye a big blue sky and every time a thought, emotion, sensation or memory arises, let it become a cloud in the sky, floating away until the next comes along. You are not your thoughts, emotions or sensations, you are the wide blue sky. Relax into that knowledge, staying here for a few minutes, peacefully watching the clouds as they come and go.

Mindfulness Jar

Seek out a clean, empty jar. Pop a tablespoon of glitter and/or stars in it, fill it two-thirds with water, add a drop or two of food colouring if you like and screw the lid on firmly. Explain to your child that they can use this jar whenever they feel jumbled up inside or when their mind is really busy. Give it a shake for a moment, then hold the jar still and watch as the sparkling contents whirl about and slowly settle. The glitter is just like our thoughts, sometimes jumbled and busy, sometimes calm and still. It is all ok. When we sit still, relax into our breathing and watch our thoughts, the mind slows and settles down too, just like the glitter in the jar. When we feel shaken up it can be hard to know what to do. When the mind is calm it is easier to work out the solutions to our problems or talk about what is upsetting us. Use the Mindfulness Jar whenever you'd like to feel calm.

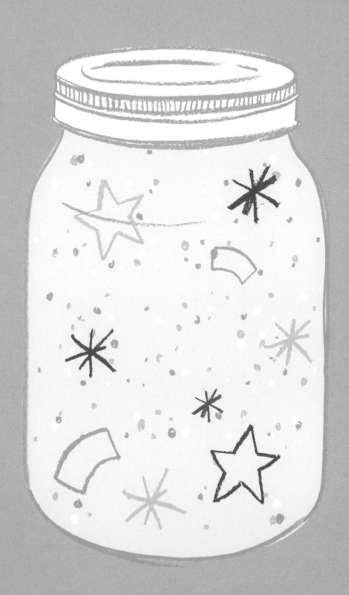

Yoga for mindfulness

Every yoga pose presents an opportunity to cultivate mindfulness and this is the essential element that turns yoga from just a stretching exercise into a mind-body well-being practice. While yoga is commonly perceived as exercise, it is much more than this. It is the anchoring of awareness on the breath or the physical sensations of the poses that makes it a mindfulness meditation practice. Approach all the yoga in the book with this quality of awareness.

ABC of mindfulness

Here is a quick step-by-step guide to cultivating mindfulness. Use this to navigate tricky thoughts, feelings or situations:

A few deep breaths, don't do anything, just feel your breathing.

B ecome aware of what is going on around you and what is happening within you – your heart rate, how your body and breathing feel, any thoughts or emotions arising. Acknowledge that these things are happening, whether they are pleasant or unpleasant, and see if you can just allow them to happen. Accept that in this moment, this is how it is.

C hoose how you respond, if you need to respond. Curiosity, compassion and sometimes comedy can be useful at this step too.

Tending to your "mind garden"

This exercise is about choosing how you focus your mind and the kind of thoughts you entertain. While it is ok to think any thought, it's important to recognize that you have a choice. You can direct your mind to thoughts that are constructive and helpful, rather than dwell on ones that bring you down. Imagine that there is a garden in your mind. Each thought that comes up is a plant emerging from the earth. The time you spend focusing on that thought is like watering that plant, directing the rays of sunshine to tend to it. Choose to direct your attention to the plants that you want to see flourish rather than nurturing those that you don't want to encourage. Be aware of the time you spend engaging in particular trains of thought and remember to lovingly tend to the flowers of your choosing. Every time you find yourself watering another plant, just notice it and bring the flow of the water back to where you want to direct it. See how things bloom as a result of your conscious choice and heart-felt energy.

Use the mantra "*I soften into this moment*"

This helps us tap into a state of mindfulness, and greater peace and ease. Remind yourself: *Don't believe everything you think!* A thought is just a thought, a passing state, not a fact.

Colour a mantra or mandala

This is for kids and adults alike. Giving the activity your full attention, purposefully choose the colours, notice the sensation of each pencil against the paper and how it feels in your hand, tune into the sound of the pencil strokes and enjoy the opportunity to express yourself. If you'd like more creative freedom, draw instead of colour in. The choice is yours!

BUILDING YOUR EMOTIONAL FIRST AID KIT

We have creams for grazes, ice for bruises and plasters for cuts. Equally we need tools to soothe emotional hurt, helping our children accept, identify and manage their emotions. Emotional first aid is a little different to dealing with physical hurt. When there's a bruise, graze or cut, our job is to relieve pain, promote healing and essentially to fix what's been damaged. With emotions, it's not about a quick fix.

I remember vividly my daughter coming home from school aged five, inconsolable that her best friend was leaving the school. My first instinct as a parent was to want to immediately take away her pain, to stop her from crying, to quickly "fix" her and help her feel happy again. In that moment, I realized that while my intentions were good, I could be doing her a disservice. Her emotional response to her friend leaving was completely normal, there was nothing unnatural about those emotions. But she needed support in managing and moving through them. Of course she would feel sad and it was not my job to deny her the right to feel sad. Emotional first aid in that circumstance was about bearing witness to my daughter's feelings first, letting her know that it was normal and that it would pass, providing a safe place to talk through her thoughts and emotions, and then looking for the presence of other feelings, such as gratitude for that friendship. When she was feeling better we tried some yoga poses to soothe her and sat down to write about how she could maintain her connection with her friend. We added to this toolkit when she was feeling sad about the loss of her grandfathers and again when she spoke of missing her grandmother who lives on the other side of the world. This is practical emotional first aid, validating your child's emotions first, empowering them with the tools to feel what they feel, to give voice to it, move through it and then take any required action to soothe or improve a situation.

coping skills

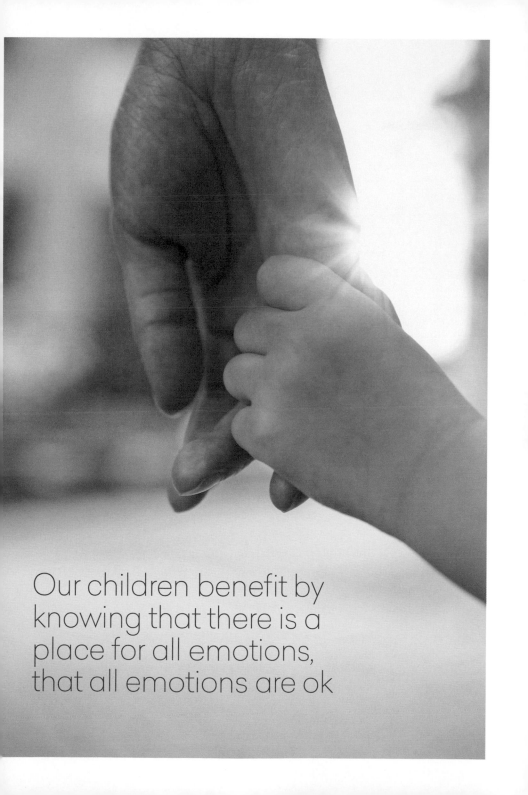

Our children benefit by knowing that there is a place for all emotions, that all emotions are ok

TALKING ABOUT EMOTIONS

The language we use around feelings is important. Often we label emotions as good or bad and this can have an impact on how we experience them and how we feel about ourselves as a result. Our children benefit by knowing that there is a place for all emotions, that all emotions are ok. While some emotions feel comfortable and pleasant, others can feel difficult and painful. They are all normal and allowing ourselves to feel the whole gamut of emotions is healthy. Mindfulness gives us the choice of what we do with them. It's important not to eradicate any emotion, because suppression generally serves to amplify them; either they leak out or we erupt like Vesuvius at an inopportune moment. Denying our emotions or the emotions of others can also result in a raft of conditions: digestive problems, heart conditions, high blood pressure, physical pain, tension, anxiety and depression. What's more useful than labelling emotions as "good" or "bad", or trying to amplify just the pleasant, is asking whether our emotions are appropriate or useful and how they can be safely expressed. This is what we explore in our emotional first aid kit.

WHAT ARE EMOTIONS & WHAT'S THEIR PURPOSE?

Emotions are messages, inviting us to take a look and see whether some action is required – every emotion is useful in this sense. The key is to understand that emotions are just signals, they're not always the gospel truth, so we need to check in and use our discernment. Is this sadness or something else? Even if we know we feel a certain emotion, we still need to enquire whether it is an appropriate response to the circumstance and one that will help us achieve our desired outcome. Remember that emotions are transient, and we can also experience several at once, so encourage curiosity.

Different emotions communicate different things to us, giving us an opportunity to stop, reflect and choose what we do with them. It's helpful to know the purpose of different emotions:

Anger arises when we feel threatened, blocked or unfairly treated. It gives us courage and prepares us to defend ourselves and those in our care.

Embarrassment is a signal that we've made an error and that some kind of correction is needed.

Anxiety alerts you to potential danger.

Guilt suggests we have broken our moral code and need to adjust our behaviour or make amends.

Doubt prompts us to take a look and assess our skills and work on any areas of weakness.

Sadness calls to us to slow down, reflect and take time out to conserve energy.

Loneliness is a signal that we need social connection.

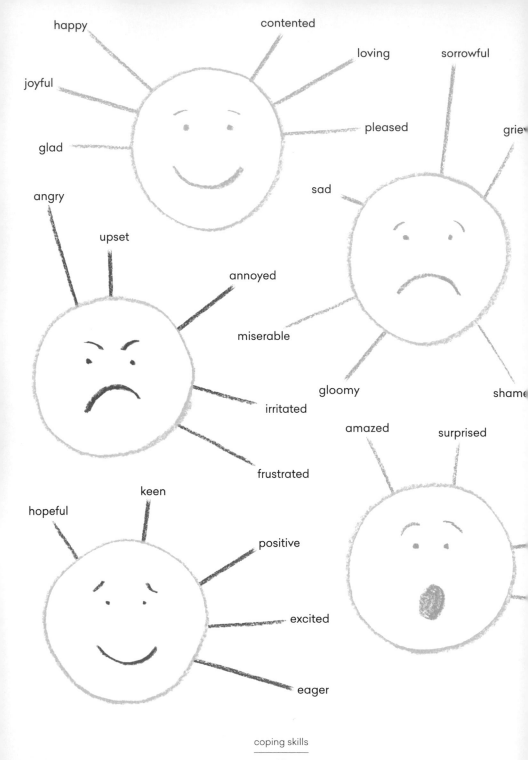

happy

contented

loving

sorrowful

joyful

pleased

grie

glad

sad

angry

upset

annoyed

miserable

gloomy

shame

irritated

frustrated

amazed

surprised

keen

hopeful

positive

excited

eager

Sit down with your child, look at the diagram of emotions opposite and talk about some of them.

When you look at the diagram, you might be surprised at just how many different types of emotions there are. Our goal is to boost our children's emotional literacy, give them a broad vocabulary of emotions and the ability to identify what it is they are feeling. Research suggests that people who can clarify and distinguish between emotions cope better in stressful situations and when angry. In one study people who could label their feelings using rich vocabulary were found to be 40 per cent less verbally and physically aggressive than those who had a tough time working out what they felt[1].

Once we can successfully identify and articulate how we are feeling, then we need to work on strategies for moving through our emotions. This is how we develop our children's emotional agility – their ability to label, accept and act on their emotions in a healthy way. Mindfulness is absolutely key to this process.

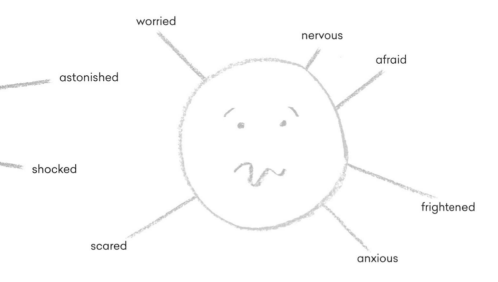

Practice: a step-by-step guide to feeling your emotions

Help your child to become aware of their emotions and make space for them. Notice how stifling an emotion can make it leak out somewhere else. Every emotion has its place and feelings can change quickly. Remember you are not your emotions. You feel it, rather than you are it.

» Can you name it?

» Where is it in your body?

» Can you describe it in words?

» Can you draw it?

» Could you describe it as a shape, colour or type of weather? Or try Professor Lea Waters' suggestion to describe an emotion as a type of animal[2].

» Can you feel it changing? What happens when you breathe a bit deeper and just watch what's happening inside?

» Can you sit with it like a friend, without wanting it to be different or wanting it to stop? Notice what happens when you let it be, when you get curious about it.

» What does it want you to do or does it have any messages for you?

» What can you do? How will you express what you are feeling? What action might you take that's helpful in this situation? It might be talking about it, writing a letter, recording it in your Self-Care Journal or using your breath or your body to help you feel better. Moving your body can be a powerful way to shift how you are feeling, so try some of the yoga in this book and see how it feels for you. The toolkits will direct you to yoga poses useful for managing specific emotions.

CULTIVATE YOUR GROWTH MINDSET

Our approach to learning, making mistakes and beliefs about our ability can play a huge role in our performance, staying power, enjoyment and self-esteem. Our children take our lead on this so actively role-modelling and helping our children develop what Carol Dweck calls a "growth" rather than a "fixed" mindset can be transformative[3]. Someone with a growth mindset sees themselves as having skills and attributes that can change and develop, while a person with a fixed mindset sees their personal qualities as unchangeable. Developing a growth mindset will help your child maximize their potential, build on their natural strengths, work on those qualities that don't come as naturally and boost their resilience in the face of failure and setbacks.

How do we build a growth mindset? Encourage your kids to allow themselves to be a beginner. You don't have to master things first go; get curious, go gently on yourself and know that there is time to grow and develop. For starters, we should watch out for the language we use verbally and internally around our skills and performance and that of others.

Instead of...	Say
"I can't"	"I am learning to" or "I am building the muscle to do this"
"I can't tie my shoelaces"	"I can't tie my shoelaces yet"
"I am rubbish at maths"	"I need to give myself time to think when I see a maths problem. When I slow down and take a few deep breaths I can see where to start and, if I get stuck, I can ask for help."
"I have awful handwriting"	"I am working on my writing"

coping skills

When it comes to mistakes, don't interpret them as evidence of your lacking in character or ability; see mistakes as an opportunity to improve, grow and learn. Effort and commitment are more important than flawless outcomes. If one strategy doesn't work, what else can you try? When you're faced with a challenge and feel that sensation of "brain squeeze", reframe this as "your brain is growing". Research clearly shows the brain has plasticity well into adulthood[4] and your child's brain is even more malleable. Share with your children that this feeling is totally normal and adults also experience it.

Our children will naturally develop a growth mindset when we praise them for their efforts, persistence, tenacity, creativity, resourcefulness and for being courageous when it comes to trying and risking a mistake, and by drawing their attention to just how far they've come. A lovely way to reconnect with them at the end of a day is to ask them, "what new strategies have you tried?" or "what did you try hard at today?"

Mantras to build a growth mindset:

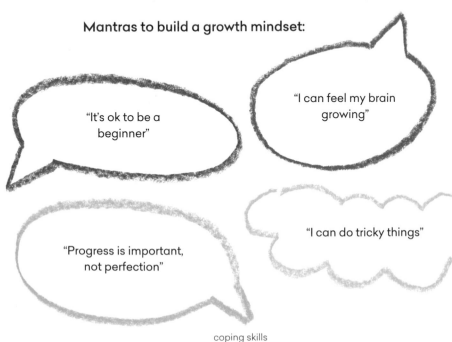

"It's ok to be a beginner"

"I can feel my brain growing"

"Progress is important, not perfection"

"I can do tricky things"

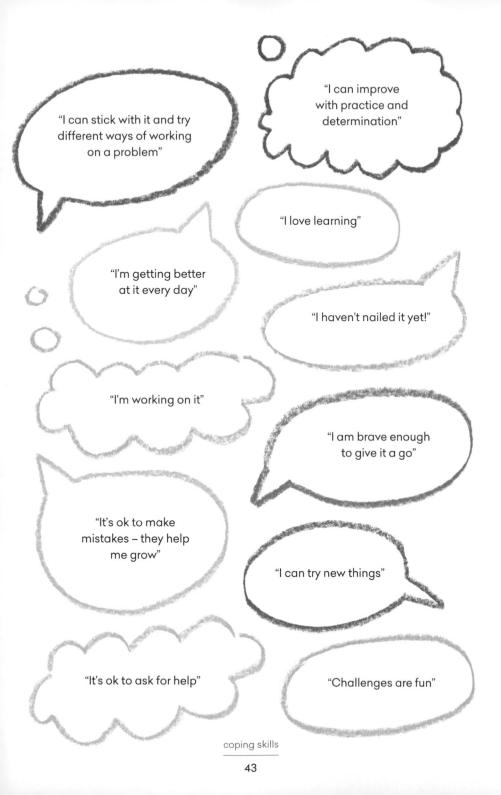

YOGA POSES TO HELP US COPE

SURFER POSE

Purpose: to build the skill of mindfulness and to tap into inner strength.

Stretch your arms out by your sides at shoulder height and step your feet wide apart so they are roughly beneath your hands. Turn your right toes out and your left heel away from you. As you breathe in, reach your arms up above your head. As you breathe out, bend your right knee deeply and bring your arms level with your shoulders. Repeat this six times, heating your body and limbering your joints. On the last repetition, stay in the lunge.

Notice how this feels for your body – what can you feel working? Do you notice your arms and shoulders? Can you feel your front thigh working hard? After a few breaths holding the pose, notice if you start to label your experience of this work... is it tough, does your inner dialogue become negative, do you want to get out of it? For another few breaths see if you can just surrender to the sensation of your body working hard, letting it be as it is, reminding yourself these feelings will pass quickly.

Come out of the lunge, give your legs a shake and try the same exercise to the other side, again noticing your reactions to how it feels. Practise allowing the sensations just to be as they are and notice how this can take some of the edge off it. The feelings are still there but the way we experience them changes. You may have also noticed that it was hard to think about other things while you were concentrating on the pose. Yoga can be a wonderful distraction when your thinking gets sticky.

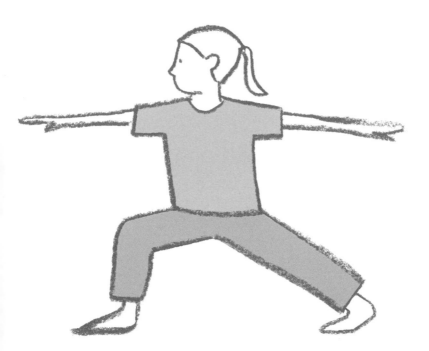

STAND TALL LIKE A MOUNTAIN

Purpose: to energize, uplift and boost confidence and courage.

Stand upright with your feet hip-width apart. Place your arms down by your sides and gaze forward. As you breathe in, raise your arms out to your sides and reach them overhead. Gaze up and press your palms together. As you breathe out, lower your arms down by your sides, elevating the crown of your head and look forward. Focus all your attention on how it feels to be moving, keeping your mind anchored on this present moment. Repeat this arm movement with your breath six times, noticing how it helps you breathe deeply and how you feel when you breathe better. On the last repetition, hold the pose with your arms overhead for a few breaths, feeling the length of your spine, the strength of your legs and tummy. Notice the sense of power, energy and focus you feel when you reach up and stand tall like a mountain.

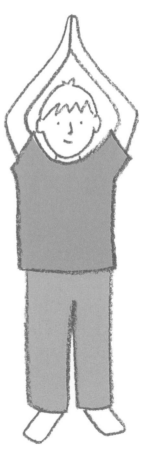

ROARING LION

Purpose: to let go of anger and things that are hard to express.

Come down to all fours. As you breathe in, look forward, draw your shoulders down from your ears and lift up your tail. As you exhale, round your spine with your chin to your chest, point your tail down, stick out your tongue and roar like a lion. Repeat this six times, feeling it release any anger or other emotion you'd like to let go of.

After Roaring Lion, you might want to relax by enjoying a few calming breaths in Ladybird pose (see page 68).

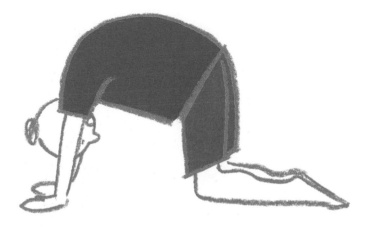

When I feel angry I will...

» Take a moment. It's ok. It will pass. I don't have to do anything right now. Pause and consider. There's real wisdom in counting to ten.

» Remember, anger is just a feeling. Use the words "I feel angry right now" rather than "I am so angry". It is not who I am, it is a passing experience. It's not bad to feel angry, it's what I do with it that matters.

» Am I "hangry"? Make sure I'm fed and watered so I can think straight.

» Consciously relax my hands, shoulders, eyes, brow and jaw. When my body is calm it is harder to feel angry.

» Breathe through it. Try the "inhale, pause, exhale, pause" (see page 66) with my hands opening and closing or get down on all fours and roar it out with Roaring Lion (see page 47).

» Move through it. Try the Surfer Pose (see page 44) to feel courageous and stand up for myself or just lie down in Resting Snowflake (see page 71). Research shows that simply lying down can reduce feelings of anger and hostility[5]. Doing this pose on a regular basis can help me feel less reactive.

» Seek out nature and notice anything I find soothing or awe-inspiring.

» Talk to myself as I would my best friend. If my best friend had gone through the same experience, what would I say to them?

» Write about it on a piece of paper, rip it up and toss it away.

» Talk about it, give voice to my feelings and don't stuff it down. It is very healing to be heard.

» Express anger the right way: keep it specific to behaviour rather than targetting the person. Avoid personal jibes about character such as "You're a nasty person". Let them know the specific action that caused my anger. (This is an important one for parents...rather than condemning our kids as "naughty", get clear on the behaviour that was out of line. We want our children to feel guilt for doing a bad thing, rather than feeling shame for being a bad person.)

» For adults or older kids: ask myself, "Is my anger helping or harming the situation?" Get perspective. Leave the room if I have to.

» For parents feeling frustrated by their kids: check in with age-appropriate behaviour and make sure I am being realistic. It may still be irritating but if I find myself thinking "Stop acting like a child"...remember, they are a child. (Guilty as charged.)

» In the heat of the moment, remember my values. What's important to me as a person, as a member of this family? Try to take action in accordance with those qualities.

» Ask myself, what lies beneath this anger? It's seldom anger on its own and if we want to move through it we need to address the cause. Am I feeling threatened, hurt, afraid, in pain, overstimulated, frustrated or fatigued? Dig a little deeper with compassion, then take action.

» Once the heat of my anger has passed, what can I do? What course of action will help me achieve my desired outcome?

» After angry episodes, try some journalling – What am I learning? What can I do differently next time? Use my writing to reaffirm how I want to behave.

When I feel hurt I will...

» Tell someone.

» Be still.

» Know that it's ok to cry.

» Rest.

» Try to calm my mind and relax my body. I could use my Mindfulness Jar or flip through my Self-Care Journal.

» Ask for a hug.

» Be gentle on myself.

» Remind myself that my feelings matter.

» Repeat to myself: *"I am safe, I am loved, I am held"*.

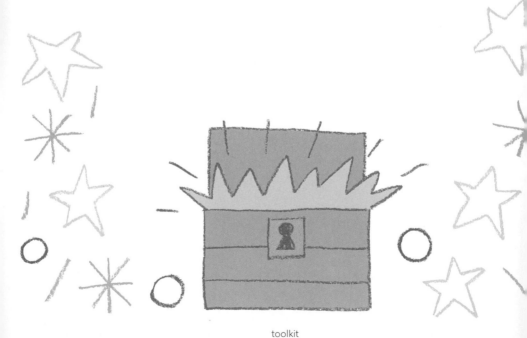

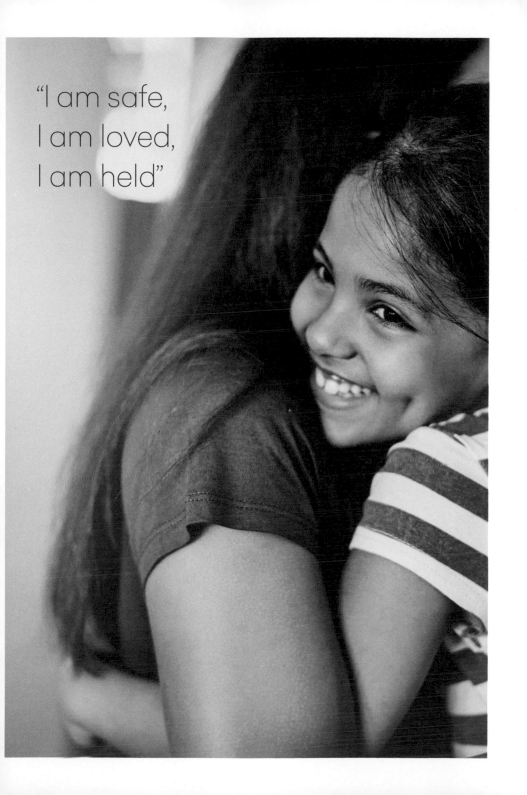

"I am safe,
I am loved,
I am held"

Calm, safe-place guided meditation script

This is just an example of a visualization you can share with your child. Create your own based on your favourite places:

Take my hand, we are going to wander down to the beach together. Slip off your shoes and feel the warmth of the soft sand beneath your feet. It is a lovely summer's afternoon and the blue sky is dotted with puffy white clouds. The day is very still, barely a breeze and the water is calm. Look out and see the sunlight glinting on the surface of the gentle waves. As we walk closer to the water's edge, notice the sand becoming firmer and cooler underfoot. Pause and take a moment to write in the sand, where the ocean laps the shore, any worries or concerns you are carrying. Watch as the little waves wash them away – the ocean can hold them for you. It's ok to release your worries. Notice how it feels to let them go. If they linger, know you can always give voice to them with me and I will help you.

Gaze out to sea. Can you taste the salty air? Who else is here with us today? Sometimes there are dolphins playing together in the waves. If we're lucky we might even see a whale breach. Look out for pelicans in flight or the old white sea eagle wheeling far out to sea. There are always cheeky seagulls to chase.

Now we walk along the water's edge toward the rock pools. Let's see what we can find today. There might be starfish, shells, brightly coloured fish darting about, maybe even a hermit crab. What can you see?

As we stand with the waves lapping at our feet, notice the sound of the birds beginning their ritual of roosting for the approaching evening in the tall trees behind you. Hear them happily squawking to each other, snuggling in with their loved ones, a deep sense of safety as they settle for the night. This is a calm, safe place.

We head back to the warm, soft sand and take a seat together. Feel my arm draped around your shoulder, drawing you near. The sun is now setting and the white clouds are turning a milky pink. The whole sky is turning a golden pink, mirrored by the surface of the water, the colour of love. The chorus of the birds is getting louder as the day is drawing to a close. Feel the deep peacefulness of this place and know that you can come here any time you want. Feel the warmth of my embrace, wrapping you up in my care. Everything is ok as it is.

TWO

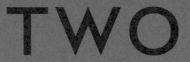

SLEEP, RELAX
& BREATHE

This chapter is all about soothing practices that promote better sleep for the whole family, and help us feel calm throughout our day. Good sleep is such a cornerstone of health but, try with all our might, we can't make sleep happen for anyone in the family, even ourselves. That's why you'll find a focus on relaxation and breathing in this chapter, in addition to tips on sleep. Modern life is full of stimulation and busyness, even for our little ones. Sleep, relaxation and being with the breath all help to mediate the effects of stress, promoting the "rest and digest" part of the nervous system. So the mantra is, *"If I can't sleep, then I will rest. If I can't stop and rest, I will feel my breath"*. There is always a way that we can soothe and calm ourselves. We want our babies to self-soothe – this is just as vital throughout the course of your whole life.

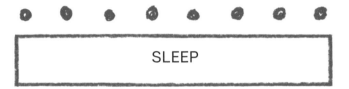

SLEEP

The quality of our sleep has a significant impact on every layer of our well-being – from our immune function, nervous system, cellular repair and growth, to our mood, focus, ability to think straight, memory, sense of humour... My mantra is *"Sleep for sanity"* and I think this resonates for every parent. It is important to recognize that, while we can't make anyone sleep, we can promote a positive relationship with sleep, we can role-model healthy sleeping habits and we can commit to healthy choices in a pre-bedtime routine that promotes our chances of good sleep. Everyone in the family benefits from having a toolkit of things to try when sleep feels elusive and anxiety kicks in.

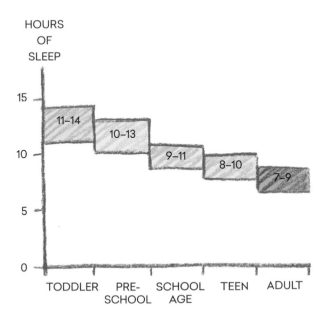

sleep, relax & breathe

DEVELOPING A POSITIVE RELATIONSHIP WITH SLEEP

In this day and age, sleep tends to get a terrible rap. Just look at the language we use around it – "I'll sleep when I'm dead" and "You snooze, you lose". FOMO (fear of missing out) is real. For our children, the worst punishment is being sent straight to bed. Culturally, we need to recognize the enormous value of sleep and learn to revere it! I want my children to feel that their bed is a safe place, not a punishment, and that going to sleep does not equate to missing out on the good stuff. I do my best to extol the virtues of sleep and each night, as my little ones go to bed, I reinforce that sleep is the thing that allows them to engage in life with full vigour: to grow, to play, to focus and have the most fun! "Happy sleep" are the last words I whisper as I kiss them goodnight. I know that I am best placed to weather the inevitable stresses of my children's bedtime when I am well slept myself, so I prioritize my opportunity for sleep too, recognizing my own individual sleep needs. My kids will also see me roll out my yoga mat or lie down with my legs up the wall after an interrupted night's sleep because we can compensate for it with soothing activities. They often join me in those nourishing practices.

TIPS TO PROMOTE BETTER SLEEP

The ideal environment for sleep is one that is dark and cool. If your child needs a night light, opt for a blue one. Keep it dimly lit, even during night wake-ups and trips to the bathroom. As much as possible, keep bedrooms clean and uncluttered, feeling like a safe haven and a place to relax, especially the area around the bed. Consistency of bedtime and rise time also helps the body clock.

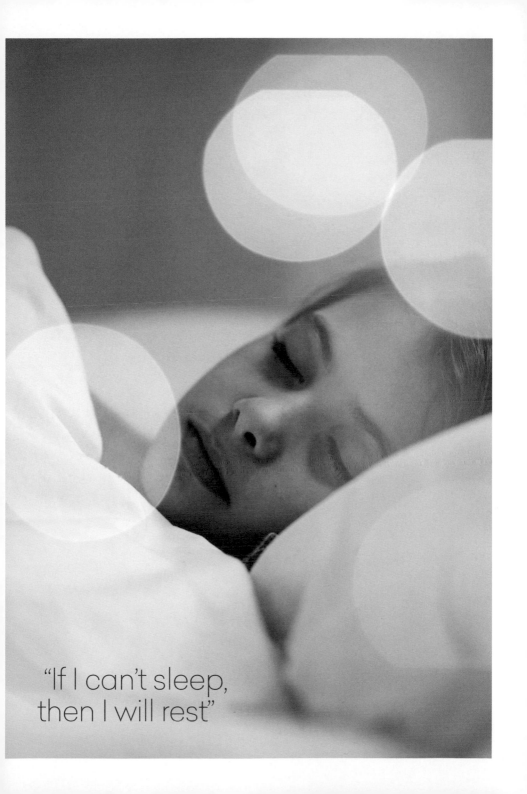

"If I can't sleep,
then I will rest"

Practice: Build your own pre-bedtime ritual

Regularity helps and mindfully engaging in soothing activities prior to bedtime can have a significant impact on feeling ready for sleep. These practices prime the mind and body for sleep and the repetition will help your child relax into knowing what comes next. Each activity also presents a little fun of its own.

» **Bathtime.** Add some children's Epsom salts or magnesium flakes; these can aid physical relaxation. For adults, try some magnesium oil spray after bathing. I recommend applying it to the feet so it doesn't tingle too much. This oil always helps me sleep better.

» **Pop on jammies you love.** Don't underestimate the power of favourite PJs.

» **Have a stretch.** Try the yoga poses on pages 68–71 or just listen to your body and tend to anything that is calling to you. Seated, all-fours and lying-down stretches are best for this end of the day, helping to quieten the mind. During your stretches, focus on making your exhalation long and smooth.

» **Hop into bed and read something soothing or listen to relaxing music or a guided meditation.** Avoid screen time in the 30 minutes prior to bedtime – it's overstimulating, scuppers your ability to get to sleep and affects the quality of your sleep.

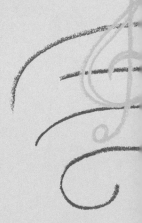

» **Spritz a little "happy dream spray" with a soothing scent on the pillow or cuddly toys.** It works for adults too. Try lavender or whatever you personally find relaxing. Buy one or turn it into a craft activity and make one at home with essential oils. Take a few deep, relaxing breaths and feel yourself softening into rest.

» **Allow sleep to come when it will.** Remind yourself that rest is just as good and, if you feel worried, turn to your soothing toolkit of things to try until sleep comes (see page 72). Remember the mantra: *"If I can't sleep, it's ok, I will rest"*.

» **Remember that good sleep doesn't have to be in one uninterrupted stretch.** Don't worry if you wake up. Try not to look at the clock or count your hours of sleep. Just soften into knowing that rest will replenish you and sleep will return. Say the words, "Sleep is coming".

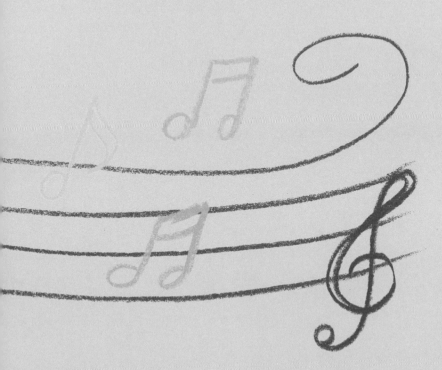

sleep, relax & breathe

RELAXATION

The ability to relax is an important skill to cultivate, helping us regulate our mood, physical comfort, energy levels and responses to challenging experiences. We need regular opportunities to release physical tension and soothe the mind, with what I call little "micro moments" of calm dotted through our day. When we get skilled at relaxing throughout the course of our day, we tend to sleep better at night too. In the absence of good sleep or during stressful times, rest and relaxation become even more important, helping us cope and heal.

WHAT IS RELAXATION?

Relaxation has both a mental and physical element. It is a state of ease, a softening and releasing, an absence of effort and striving. It can be in stillness or we can experience a state of relaxation in gentle movement too. Relaxation doesn't have to take a lot of time, it can be as short as feeling the sensation of a few deep breaths or watching the moving clouds for a minute. Alternatively, we can set aside time for a longer restorative practice with activities such as meditation, guided visualizations or soothing yoga.

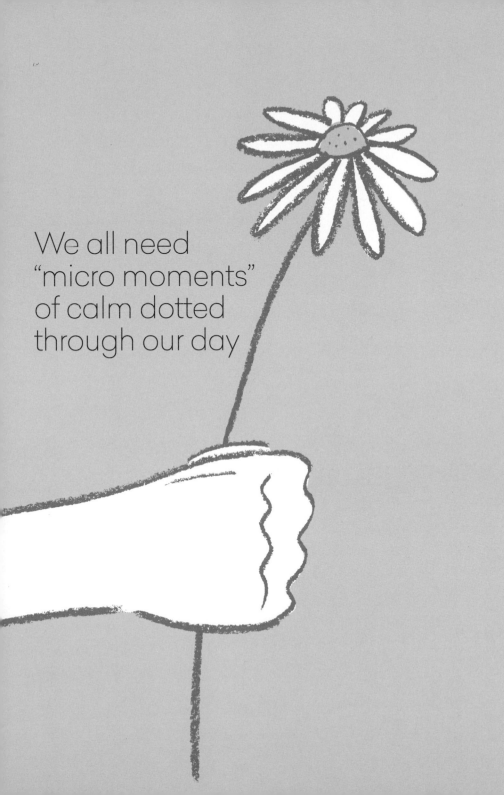

We all need
"micro moments"
of calm dotted
through our day

Practices to cultivate relaxation

What is tension and what is relaxation?

Sometimes we hold on to physical tension without even realizing it. This sequential "squeeze and relax" exercise will help you know the difference. Guide your child through this exercise, working with the breath for older children or just focusing on squeezing the body part for younger kids.

» Lie on your back with your arms by your sides and take a moment to notice how your whole body feels.

» Starting with your hands, as you exhale, squeeze them into a tight fist. As you breathe in, relax them.

» As you breathe out, bend your arms, squeeze your biceps and make a fist. Breathe out and relax.

» Breathe in and tense your arms and hands and squeeze your shoulders up to your ears. Exhale, let go.

» Inhale and squeeze your arms, hands and shoulders and scrunch up your face. Exhale and enjoy the release.

» Breathe in and squeeze your arms, hands, shoulders, face, chest and tummy. Exhale and soften it all.

» Inhale and squeeze your arms, hands, shoulders, face, chest, tummy and the whole length of your legs, flexing your heels. Exhale, let it all go and soften into the sensation of your body resting on the floor, the breath moving through your body.

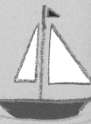

» Notice how different you feel now.

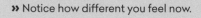

Relaxation on the go

Try some "chicken wing" shoulder rolls. Breathe in, bend your arms like a wing, lift your elbows up and out to your sides. Breathe out, draw your elbows back and down. Repeat six times and try to lift the crown of your head too, to feel more alive. Or try some "yoga of the face": consciously soften your forehead especially between your eyebrows, relax your jaw, soften your tongue, stick it out if you want to. Return to your day with greater peace and ease.

Calming your mind with a mantra

If your mind is busy or stuck on an unhelpful thought, anchoring it on a mantra can help and you'll find lots of different ones to choose from throughout this book. With your child, make some mantras of your own. One of our favourites is by @gratefulmother: *"I am still, I am calm, I am me"*. In your Self-Care Journal, you could make some art featuring your mantras.

Soothing magic lake visualization

Lie on your back either with your legs stretched out or, if it's more comfortable, with your knees bent and feet flat on the floor. Bring your hands to gently rest on your tummy with your elbows supported by the floor. Imagine that there is a magical lake contained in your abdomen. Your fingertips are resting on the surface of the water, maybe there are ducks or little boats bobbing on the surface. Feel the soft movement of your breath as it gently moves the surface of the water and the ducks or boats floating on it. Send your mind's eye into the water. What colour is it? Is it still or are there currents? Are there fish glinting in the sunlight? Are there plants moving with the gentle ripples? How deep is it? Notice how the light filters through at the surface but, as you get deeper down, the water becomes dimly lit and very still. Imagine the silty, sandy bottom of the lake. Notice how still and calm the water is at the bottom. Let your mind's eye explore your lake – you never know what you might find! A treasure chest, sunken ship or singing mermaid. Allow your mind to rest on any part of it that you find soothing.

BREATHING

Working with your breath is a wonderful way to relax and replenish without taking much time, energy or effort. When we breathe better, we feel better, so a super-quick way to shift your mood or alleviate tension is to work with the breath. This doesn't need to be anything fancy or elaborate, just feeling the sensations of your breathing will help to regulate it.

WHAT IS BREATHING WELL?

When we are breathing well, our breath is relaxed, smooth and expansive. It's not just contained in the lungs – with the inhalation, we will feel an expansive opening in the abdomen, sides, back, chest and collar bones, and an effortless retraction back to the centre with the exhalation. You will feel movement in different areas and we are aiming for movement in all the areas I noted above, not just the chest or the belly. Often when we are stressed our breath gets held short, tight, fast and focused in the chest. To soothe, allow the breath to move into the abdomen and sides too. A smooth belly breath can alleviate feelings of anxiety swiftly. Making the exhalation longer than the inhalation will also promote a feeling of calm.

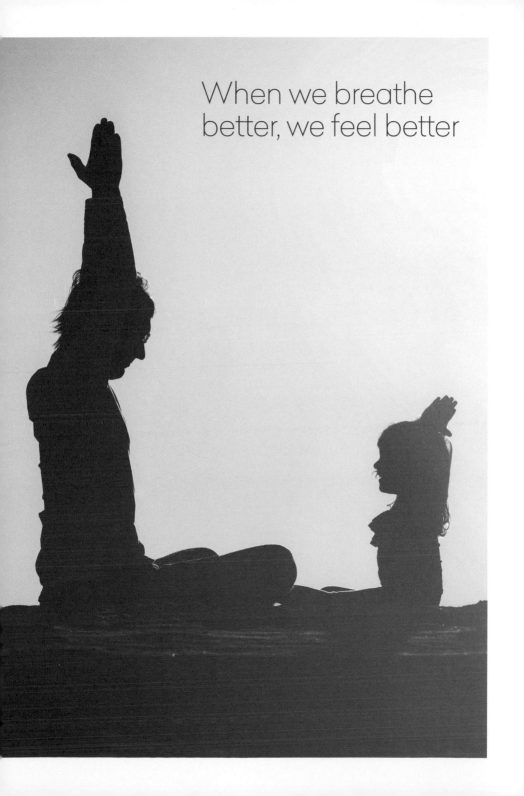

When we breathe better, we feel better

Practices to work with your breath

Balloon belly breathing

Lie on your back and rest your hands on your tummy.
Relax your body and allow your breath to be smooth.
Imagine there is a balloon in your tummy. The balloon
inflates with each breath in and gently deflates with each
breath out, your hands going along for the ride. There is
no hurry to fill or empty your balloon. See if you can take
longer to empty it than fill it back up. If you like, you could
pop a treasured cuddly toy on your tummy and watch it
ride the breath up and down. Once you've enjoyed several
relaxed deep breaths, give your toy a cuddle and feel how
much you love it. Then wrap your arms around yourself,
give yourself a tight squeeze and extend that same feeling
of love toward you.

Move your hands and feel your breath

Rather than thinking about your breathing or trying to
deepen your breath, try this simple exercise using your
hands. Sit in a relaxed position with the back of your
hands resting on your thighs. As you breathe in, stretch
your fingers out wide, opening your palms, and notice a
little pause at the end of your inhalation. As you breathe
out, make a gentle fist and notice a little pause at the
end of your out breath. Repeat this ten times, feeling how
the movement of your hands is mirrored by your whole
ribcage and tummy. Stretching open the palms actually
opens up your body to receive a more expansive in breath
and making a fist helps to engage your tummy muscles,
emptying the lungs more completely. Notice how this
happens on its own without you having to make it happen.
Feel how there is a real sense of peace in that little pause
at the end of the inhalation and the end of the exhalation.
Notice how calm the mind becomes as the breath
becomes smoother and longer.

Playing with the breath

~~~~~~~~~~

To encourage an awareness of breathing and a nice long exhalation, try blowing bubbles outside or create your own origami windmill and make it turn with your breath. Purse your lips and see how smooth you can make your breath. Imagine you are very gently blowing out a candle – how delicately can you blow?

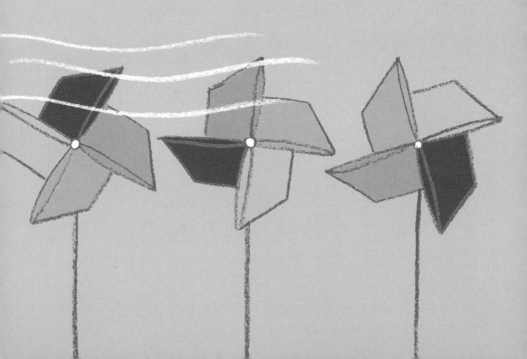

YOGA POSES TO SOOTHE AND CALM

LADYBIRD

Purpose: to calm your mind and body.

Begin on all fours with your knees hip-width apart. As you breathe out, sink your bottom to your heels and bring your forehead down onto the floor. Bring your arms like a ladybird's wings, one at a time, around behind you so your palms face upward beside your feet. Stay here for 5–10 long, relaxed breaths, longer if it feels really good. Notice how you can feel the breath move into your back and how calming this feels.

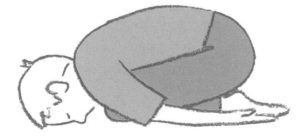

DOWNWARD DOG

Purpose: to stretch out your legs and spine.

From all fours, tuck your toes under and, as you breathe in, lift your hips up and your knees off the floor. As you breathe out, let your head hang freely and bring your heels toward the floor. Don't worry if your legs don't straighten or your heels don't touch the floor. The goal is to create an upside down "V" shape with your body and to lengthen your spine as much as possible. Hang out here for 5–10 breaths.

SLEEPING DOVE

Purpose: to relax your hips.

From all fours, bring your right knee to the floor by your right hand, slide your right foot in front of your left hip, slide your left leg further back behind you along your mat and lower your body down toward the floor, earthing your brow on the floor with your arms extended or placing your head on your folded arms. Keep your elbows wide apart to soften your shoulders. Relax the muscles of your back, bottom and thighs. Hold the pose for 5–15 breaths, then repeat on the other side.

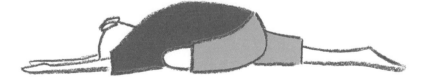

LYING DOWN TWIST

Purpose: to release your back.

Draw your knees into your chest and take your arms out wide by your sides at shoulder height. Bring your knees over toward your right elbow and relax your legs and feet completely down to the floor. Hold onto the top knee with your right hand to anchor your legs. Gaze toward the left and hold here for 5–10 breaths, letting gravity do the work for you. Repeat to the other side.

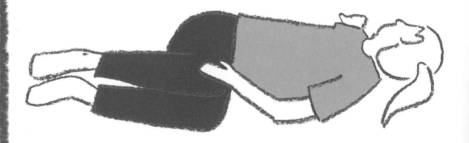

RESTING SNOWFLAKE

Purpose: to soothe and relax.

Lie down on your back with your arms loosely out by your sides, palms facing upward. Have your feet hip-width apart and let your toes drop out to the sides. Feel your whole body drop to the floor and the floor rise to meet it, feeling held by the earth. Let gravity do the work for you, weighting your body to the floor. There is nothing to be done and nowhere else to be. Enjoy the sensation of relaxing and the breath moving through your body for five minutes.

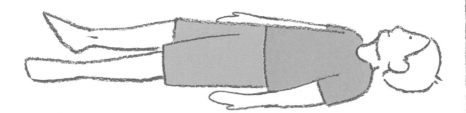

When I can't sleep, I will...

» Remind myself that it's ok. Sleep will come and until then, rest is just as good.

» Feel my breathing.

» Try the "squeeze and relax" exercise (see page 62). Once I've finished, repeat the words: "I soften into this moment".

» If it's hard to slow down my mind, I'll give it something to think about. I can either replay my day, trying to remember all the little bits, or if I choose to, focusing on the parts I enjoyed the most. Or I can create my "Best Day Ever", walking through my day from start to finish, imagining the most amazing ways to fill it, with people I'd love to share it with. I might nod off before I get to lunchtime.

» Try the "Blue Sky Mind" exercise (see page 30). Watch my thoughts, feelings, memories and sensations and imagine they are just floating clouds in a wide blue sky. Watch them come and go. I am not my thoughts, I am the wide blue sky.

» Sing a calm song.

» Repeat a mantra: *"I am calm, I am still, I am me"*.

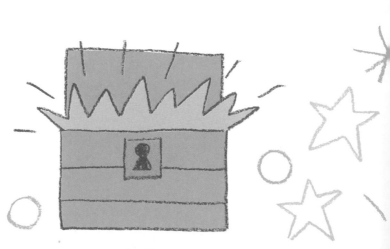

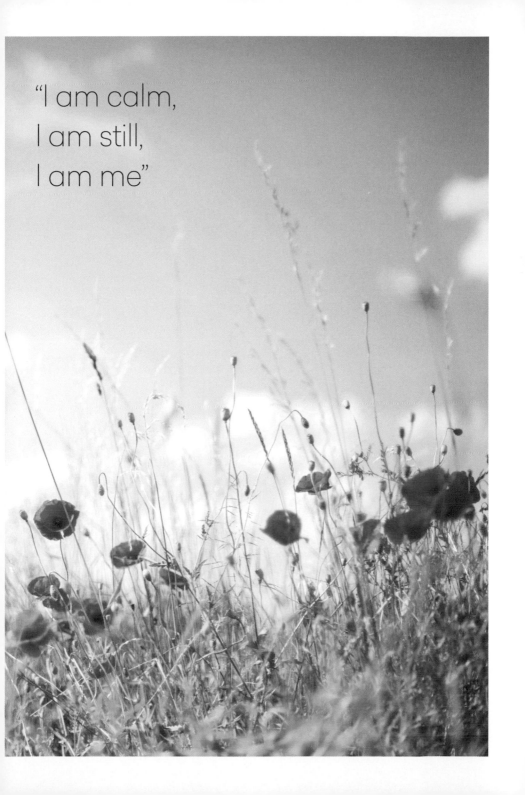

"I am calm,
I am still,
I am me"

Lying down meditation script

To calm and soothe, perfect before bed, even in bed, or whenever your child is feeling anxious:

Lie down with your arms placed by your sides, palms facing upward and your legs outstretched, toes dropping out to the sides. Wriggle the wriggles out until you feel at ease and you can let your body become really still. Relax your whole body. Let your whole body drop down deep into the support beneath you. Focus your mind on how it feels to be lying here, relaxing and letting go. Feel the back of your body sinking into the floor. Notice the sensation of your clothes against your skin.

Feel the air gently brushing the skin of your face. Soften all the muscles of your face. Relax your jaw, let go of your cheeks and lips and soften even the tongue in your mouth. Allow there to be a little space between the top and bottom rows of your teeth. Relax your eyebrows and feel as though they are gently sliding away from each other, smoothing out your forehead. Feel how relaxed your eyes are becoming – they are like pools of water, a real depth and stillness there.

Relax your neck and feel the passageways through your throat opening up to make more space for each fresh new breath that you take. Feel your head, neck and shoulders drop heavily into the floor and notice how relaxed your arms are becoming, your fingers gently curling in toward your palms as if you are holding a small, fluffy white cloud in each hand.

Travel back up through your arms and now feel your heart centre lifting and expanding, full of love. Feel your breath gently moving your chest and your tummy and deep within your tummy, notice a deep feeling of being calm and safe – this is always with you wherever you are.

Feel the whole length of your spine held by the floor, your legs, feet and toes completely relaxed. Feel all your muscles relax away from the bones and let even your bones drop. Feel how heavy your whole body has become. See if you can allow your body to feel as heavy as a stone, dropping deep into the ground beneath you. Stay with this feeling of heaviness for a few deep breaths. Now feel your body becoming lighter, maybe as light as a feather, almost as if you are floating. Stay with this sensation of lightness for a few expansive breaths. Release this feeling of lightness and notice again the sensation of your clothes against your skin and feeling each part of your body that's in contact with the floor. Feel how the earth is rising to meet you, holding you in an embrace. The earth is always there, supporting you, holding you, like my love.

(If your child is preparing for sleep, end here.)

Now gently wriggle your fingers and your toes. Feel a sense of liveliness returning to your whole body. Make any other gentle movements that call to you. Feel your sense of the here and now coming back to you. Blink your eyes open and slowly re-enter your day, feeling your calm-abiding centre, the earth beneath you, wrapped up in my love.

THREE

· · · · · · · ·

ENVIRONMENT

This spoke of the Vitality Wheel is all about
your environment and the impact it has on your
well-being, mental clarity and mood. It includes
where we live, the space we inhabit and the skin
we live in. We will also explore the therapeutic
power of being in nature, the practices that tap
into those benefits and the significance of place –
locations that anchor us in a sense of history and
personal meaning.

INSIDE ENVIRONMENT

While we all have our own individual chaos threshold, there is no denying that outer order creates inner harmony. A good vacuum will literally blow out the cobwebs in your mind. Even if you think mess doesn't bother you, notice the difference to your mood, energy and clarity of thinking after a swift tidy up. Talk about this insight with your kids. Take stock of your inside environment, your home, where you work and even your car, and notice the impact it is having on your collective well-being. How you take action is totally up to you. You can break it down and tidy up one area or room at a time, or enjoy a blitz and spend a weekend doing a "spring clean", any time of year. Developing routines or rituals that promote order will help you keep tidy and the younger you start, the more this becomes a family habit, with a sense of shared ownership.

» **Tidy-up time.** Part of just about any activity is "tidy-up time". This works when you engage in one activity at a time, rather than attempting several at once. Give one game your full attention and when interest wanes, pack away before moving on to the next. When my kids were little, they'd follow my lead and we would clear away together, making it part of the fun. Now they are older, the habit is formed and they're more capable of completing the task on their own, sometimes unprompted, sometimes with help.

» **Everything has a home.** If you want to create order and harmony in your inside environment, everything needs to have a home. Good storage is life changing. It can be as simple as plastic boxes or large storage bags all earmarked for certain contents. This will keep things neat and you'll be able to locate items with far greater ease. Be realistic about the volume of belongings that you can house in an orderly fashion. I find that my children play more happily with fewer things neatly stored and easily accessible than when we are bursting at the seams. A good cull can be deeply therapeutic. Sometimes this is better done on your own, sometimes your children will want to be involved and will feel uplifted by the act of gifting their treasured belongings to younger family members or to charity.

» **One in one out.** If space is a prized commodity, a "one in one out" policy can help. When we receive a bag of hand-me-down clothes or toys, we need to clear some space before the new items can find a home. This can become a ritual around birthdays and Christmas, clearing the decks for the new and passing on the old.

» **Daily rituals.** Often children have a genuine interest in being involved. Encourage your little ones to help you make the beds, set and clear away the table, and join in the washing up. We are all responsible for the harmony of the home environment so encourage ownership that is age appropriate and enjoy doing it together, noticing the positive impact it has on you as a family unit.

» **Make your home beautiful to you.** Encourage self-expression in your children's rooms with colours and motifs they love. It doesn't need to be grand or elaborate, simple touches can make all the difference – a poster they've made, photos of happy moments or special people, a rug they love, a comfy chair in a space flooded with natural light. Make the most of what they have and enjoy creating a space that feeds their soul.

» **Create a safe place.** Kids love making a den or hiding place. This can be a structure that's permanent or something temporary and you are limited only by your imagination.

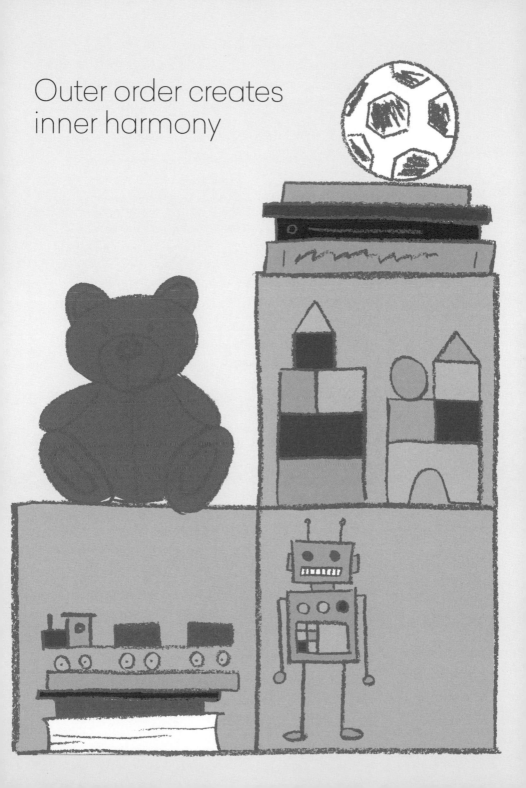

Outer order creates inner harmony

NURTURING THE SKIN YOU LIVE IN

Caring for our environment should extend to caring for our bodies – they are the outer casing that we inhabit continuously. An awareness of our body and clothing can make a world of difference to our comfort and satisfaction.

» Observe the basics of hygiene: bathing, brushing teeth and washing hair. The simple act of washing your hands can be a mindfulness practice – feeling the sensation of the water cleansing the skin, the scent of the hand gel and the feeling of any nasties being washed away. Even better, take a mindful bubble bath and let worries soak away.

» What you wear. When you have the choice, wearing colours and clothes you love can lift your mood. It's not about impressing anyone else; choose what makes you feel happy and vibrant.

» Listen to your body. Use your mindfulness skills to get quiet and really tune in. Children can be remarkably resilient, bouncing back quickly from injuries but, as a parent, I'm often surprised by the things my kids don't volunteer. Rather than wait for them to offer it up, I regularly ask them how their bodies are feeling and take action.

» Touch. There's nothing more healing than a good cuddle. Engage in regular therapeutic hugs or snuggles over stories and everyone benefits. Your little ones might enjoy gentle massage. They can lie in your lap, head cradled tenderly, while you use your fingertips like a pitter patter of rain on their foreheads. Great for soothing a worried mind.

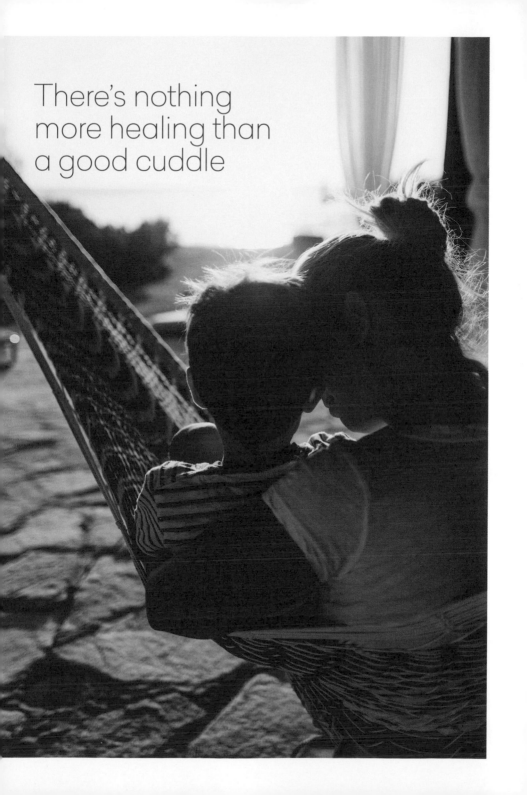

There's nothing more healing than a good cuddle

THE GREAT OUTDOORS

From as early as I can remember, nature has been a great tonic to me. I remember as a child walking with my family on the headland nature reserve in Sydney, playing on the beach making tunnels and sandcastles, swimming in the ocean pools, looking for crabs, and spotting birds around the lagoons – these were bonding activities that we all enjoyed. My brothers are nine years older than me, so these became treasured collective pursuits. As I got older, sitting on the cliffs, watching the ocean and feeling the fresh sea spray, helped me settle in preparation for exams or sporting performances. When my first little one was born, I'd bundle her into the baby carrier and take the same trails on the headland as I did when I was a child, feeling a sense that everything was going to be ok. During my father's 15-month battle with motor neurone disease, when he was no longer able to tread those paths, I would share with him all the wildlife I had seen on my walk that day, describing the conditions of the swell and the colours of the skyscape. And now that I no longer live in the environment in which I grew up, I rely on images and my own imagination to take me there. These form the basis for a soothing and grounding meditation whenever I need to feel connected. One of the most potent ways to feel settled in a new place is to connect with the environment around you. I relish walking through the woods looking for deer, a very new environment to me, but I've learned that you can be just as nourished by forest bathing as sun bathing.

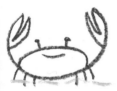

Wherever you are, you will find nature to soothe and uplift you. Having lived on the sunny beaches of Sydney, in gritty urban locations in London, and now in the rolling hills of England, I have always found something in nature to revive me. Being in nature is like hitting the reboot button, soothing us, quietening the mind and connecting us with what we feel is important in life. Research clearly shows that time spent in nature is good for collective mental and physical health[6] and that feeling disconnected from nature can lead to a wide range of behavioural problems including negative moods, attention difficulties and higher rates of physical and emotional illnesses[7]. There is even new research suggesting that time in the great outdoors can boost positive body image and a healthy respect for our bodies[8]. So get outdoors with your kids! It is free, accessible, and so easily done! Sharing with your family the things that pique your interest or things you find awe inspiring is a wonderful way to share time, drawing you close together. This can transform any moment, whether you are in the car or on foot. I love that my three-year-old has embraced this skill, pointing out a red kite on the wing or curious cloud formations. Being on the lookout for nature's beauty is the best self-care strategy on the go.

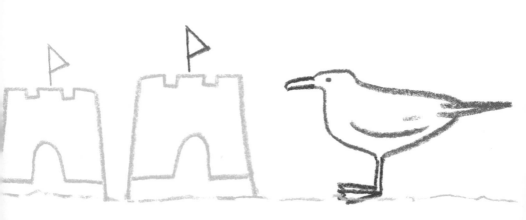

NATURE AS A METAPHOR

Mankind has always been inspired by nature. It can provide many powerful metaphors to help us navigate life. Seek out metaphors in the environment around you and share them with your kids. You might find that they draw on these symbols their whole lives. My family love that the turning seasons remind us there is a time for all things: a time for newness, a time for decay, a time for activity and effort, and a time for stillness and rest. It is a metaphor too for the passing experience of emotions in all their tones. Encourage your kids to reflect on the pleasures unique to each season, even winter! This is one of the greatest life tools – learning to embrace the beauty and the blessings around us rather than hankering for something else. We appreciate the tenacity of the daffodils emerging through the snow, the flexibility and resilience of bamboo, the weeping willow's strength and ability to regenerate, and of course we like to channel the power of standing tall like a mountain.

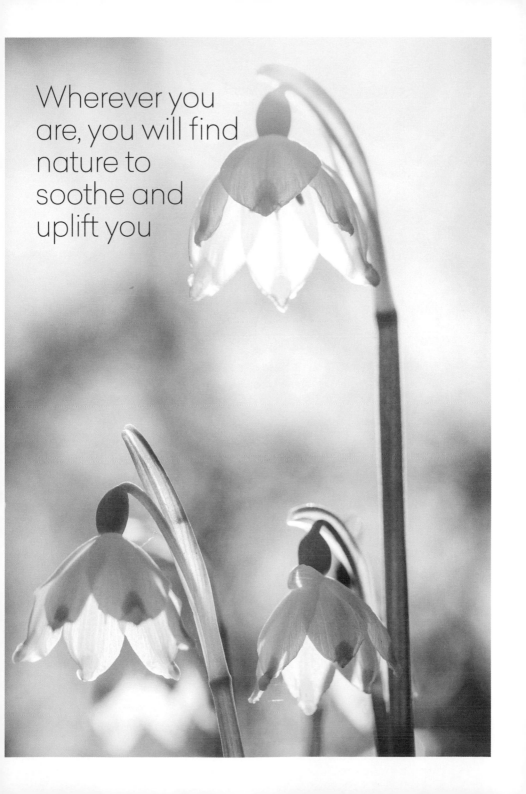

Wherever you are, you will find nature to soothe and uplift you

Practices to absorb the beauty of nature

Nature walk

Go out together with the express intention of noticing the environment around you. Make sure there are no distractions, this is just time to be absorbed by nature's beauty. Only bring out your phone to take photos. It's not a time for worry, thoughts about the "to do" list, or squabbles. Appreciate and give voice to the things you see, hear and smell, so you can all enjoy them. Notice how your environment changes with the seasons, giving you fresh inspiration throughout the year. One of my favourite mindfulness moments with my kids was engaging in an impromptu sound meditation while walking through snow, honing in on the crunch underfoot. You might be surprised by what reels you all in.

Nature count

On your walk, count all the types of flowers, plants or birds you can identify. Take a spotter's guide to broaden your knowledge. Our favourite is the bird count and we are enjoying getting to know lots of different birds in our new neck of the woods. This is a powerful mindfulness tool – keeping your mind anchored on something replenishing and building your sense of connection and belonging in your local environment. Even simpler, count the colours you see on the way or the different-shaped leaves you find.

Mini-beast hunt

Find out who lives in your garden or neighbourhood. Take a magnifying glass and have a really close look.

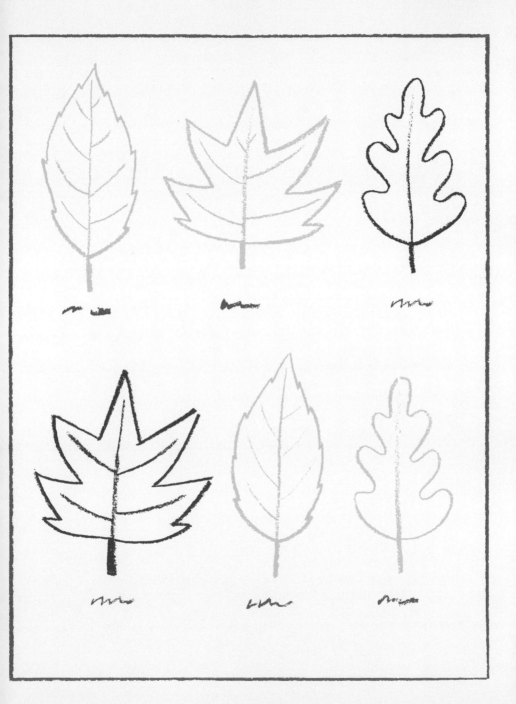

Look up!

Simply lie back and watch the moving cloudscape or the boughs of a tree, spot the planes, count the vapour trails or look for birds in flight. Have a big night out with your kids and watch the stars.

Savour a sunrise or a sunset together

A powerful way to feel a sense of gratitude and awe.

Get your hands dirty

Get stuck into the gardening, planting seeds or seedlings, weeding and pruning together or let your little ones make mud pies. Working with the soil can be a real tonic for anxiety, depression and anger.

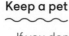

Indoor gardening

Display cut flowers or grow house plants, all of which boost collective well-being.

Encourage the local wildlife

Put out a couple of feeders and see who visits.

Keep a pet

If you don't have your own you could see if there are some neighbourhood pets that could do with some extra love and attention. Time spent looking after an animal is a potent mood booster, teaching kindness, responsibility and how to be of service to another.

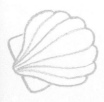

Gather some flowers and press them at home

Use a heavy book or invest in a simple flower press. These are perfect for decorating homemade cards.

Get absorbed together

Try a search for four-leaf clovers to encourage really close looking and a natural treasure hunt.

Nature art

Form mandalas on the ground and leave them for others to enjoy, make an autumn wreath, thread some daisy chains, build towers of stones, or bring leaves and shells inside to make your own creations.

Nature recordings

The documentary series *The Blue Planet* and *Planet Earth* are wonderful nature therapy resources. Nature CDs are another option, including sounds from the ocean, waterfalls, rainfall or birdsong. We love trying to work out which call belongs to which bird.

Nature bingo games

When the weather isn't inviting, we stay indoors and pull out one of these board games. You don't need to be able to read, even my three-year-old loves joining in. We started with bird bingo, branched out to cat bingo and have settled on bug bingo as the collective favourite.

SIGNIFICANT PLACES

Having just returned from a visit to my childhood home, the significance of place feels very fresh and potent to me. Just being there felt deeply healing, reminding me of anecdotes I could share with my kids to build their mental snapshot and connection with family members who had come before them. There are some places that are etched into the cells and fibres of your body and being there makes you feel like you have plugged into the flow of life itself. These may be places where you grew up or places you visited with special people, somewhere connected with some kind of special memory or just an aspect of the environment that speaks deeply to you. Sharing these places with those you love can be profoundly bonding and energizing, building a sense of shared history, meaning and lineage.

Where are the places that feel resonant for you and your family? Are there particular environments that make you feel alive? Is there a place you like to go to remember someone? I feel more connected with my father when walking on a beach or watching a bird on the wing than I do by his graveside. This is deeply personal so reflect on the places of most meaning for you. If you can't get to the places you hold dear, I appreciate that this can be painful. Try building new places of significance, visit brand-new locations or pretend you are a tourist in areas closer to home and see life with fresh eyes.

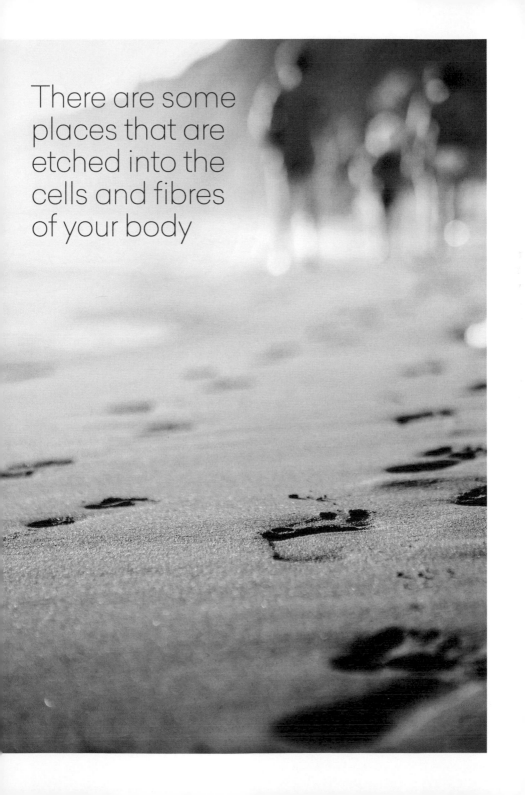

There are some places that are etched into the cells and fibres of your body

TREE POSE

Purpose: to stand your ground and feel focused.

Begin with your feet hip-width apart. Take your right big toe to the instep of your left foot, or plant the sole of your right foot against your inner calf or thigh of the left leg. Fully straighten the left leg, take the right knee out wide and angle it straight down to the ground. Keep your hips and chest square. Bring your hands to your heart or extend them up and out to the sky in a "V" shape. Enjoy breathing smoothly here, focusing on elevating the crown of the head skyward as you send roots down through your standing foot. Be here and breathe, sense of humour essential! Hold for 5–15 breaths and then repeat on the other side. Try this on your own or with a helper.

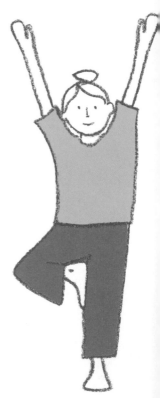

TRIANGLE TO HALF-MOON POSE

Purpose: to feel connected and energized.

Face sideward along your mat with your feet one-and-a-half times shoulder-width apart. Turn your right toes out and bring your left heel angled away from you at 45 degrees. Keeping both legs straight, hinge at your right hip and bring your right hand onto your right shin. Turn your abdomen and chest toward the sky and stack your left shoulder on top of your right, reach your left arm up to the sky. Enjoy 5–10 breaths here. Come into Half-moon pose by bending your right knee, bringing the fingertips of your right hand to the floor and seeing if you can lift your left foot off the floor – just see! Again hold for 5–10 breaths. Repeat the sequence on the other side. Parents: you can pretend to be a wall for your kids to lean into or they can be super brave and try it solo.

WEEPING WILLOW

Purpose: to let go and refresh.

Stand with your feet hip-width apart and your knees slightly bent. Drape your spine forward along your thighs and let your head and fingertips dangle toward the floor like the branches of a weeping willow. Be still or have a little sway, letting go of what you no longer need.

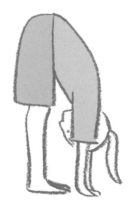

When I feel bored I will...

» Relish it! When life gets busy or the next thing is required of me, I'll crave the luxury of boredom.

» Get quiet, listen to my mind and body and notice what it is telling me. What do I need right now?

» Flip through the yoga in this book and try a pose that looks interesting to me.

» Turn to my Self-Care Journal or my Vitality Wheel for inspiration and find an activity that appeals to me.

» Ask if anyone needs help or would like some company.

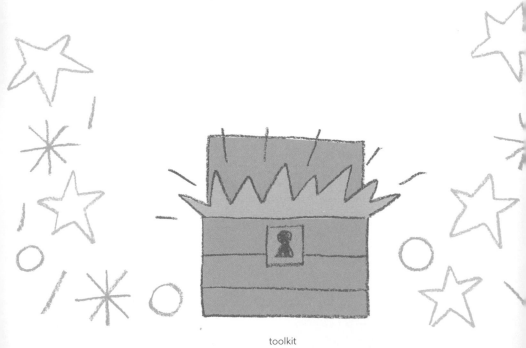

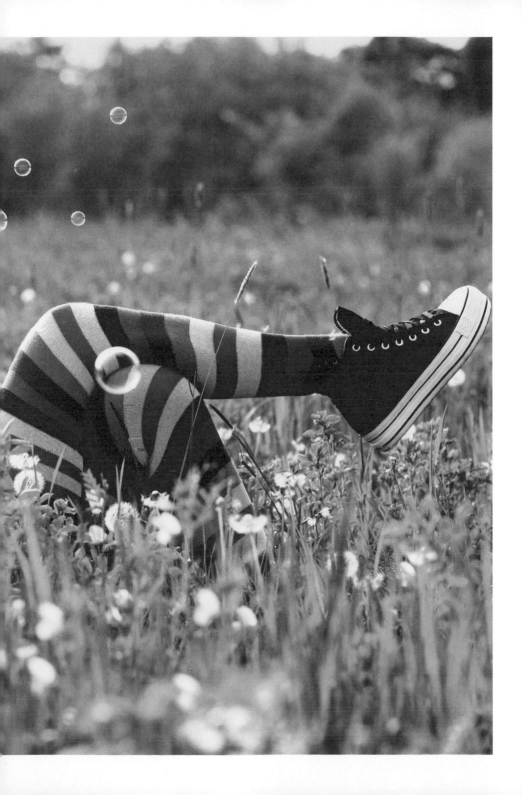

FOUR

HAPPINESS

This spoke of the Vitality Wheel is all about happiness. Before we dive in, it's important to acknowledge that the goal isn't perpetual happiness – family life is a rich tapestry of all emotions. This chapter is about empowering you with simple practices that will help shift the collective mood and lift everyone's spirits.

Every family needs a "Happiness Treasure Box" to dip into when life gets tough, tempers flare, boredom descends or just when there is time to fill. Talking about what goes into your treasure box is a joyful conversation in itself and when you have written down lots of different options you will have inspiration at your fingertips whenever you need it. Make a drawing together of all the things in your treasure box and stick it on the refrigerator for easy reference. The concept of having a treasure box is powerful because it teaches your children that happiness is not just one person, place, activity or thing, it is many. If one becomes inaccessible, you can dip into your other sources of happiness. This chapter is divided into happiness-boosting skills and happiness-boosting activities, empowering you and your kids with a potent mood booster, any time, any place.

HAPPINESS-BOOSTING SKILLS

Cultivate these skills in your children by role-modelling them, talking about them, rewarding them and building them into your rituals and core values. These skills will help you and your children see life through a fresh lens, one that promotes individual and collective well-being.

» **Savouring.** This is my all-time favourite self-care tip. It takes no real energy, effort or time and it is so powerful! Savouring is the ability to be really present to pleasurable experiences. I describe it as savouring the joyful moments of life. Build your savouring muscle by noticing moments of peace and delight, don't waste them by dividing your attention or letting your inner chatter sabotage them. You can savour the past by reminiscing about happy memories. You can savour the present by giving this moment your full attention and using all your senses to amplify the feelings of joy. You can savour the future by anticipating events to come. Teach your kids the art of savouring and they will have access to happiness in any moment. Savour with your kids and you'll have many treasured moments bonding you together.

» **Kindness and compassion.** A giant dollop of kindness and compassion transforms the most challenging of times. Feeling a sense of shared humanity is a cornerstone of collective well-being. Being of service to others deepens our bonds, roots us firmly in perspective, seeing clearly those that have less than us, and boosts both mood and self-esteem. Seeking kinder attributions for the behaviour of others gives us greater flexibility in how we respond to them. Look for ways to be kind to others and see how this transforms your day. Extending those same feelings toward ourselves alleviates internal pressure and lifts negativity.

To tap into compassion for older children, share with them the concept of the "inner elder". Move over inner critic, let the inner elder have the microphone. Your inner elder is ready and waiting to offer kind words of support, empathy and encouragement. This can either be their future grey-haired self, or an internalized voice of someone trusted, such as a grandparent. In moments of struggle and self-criticism, ask them to stop and tune in to what their inner elder would have to say.

» **Teach your children about the power of their words.** What they say about themselves out loud and their inner dialogue is important. It's an error to think that being hard on ourselves creates a better outcome – kindness, in my experience, always coaxes a better, more life-giving result. Often our children's inner dialogue is created by the voices of their parents. Be mindful of what you role-model as an individual here and be conscious of shaping their actions with kind words. Of course there is room for evaluation of behaviour but done with tenderness and restraint. To shape kinder inner dialogue, use the mantra: *"Only talk to yourself as*

A giant dollop
of kindness and
compassion
transforms the
most challenging
of times

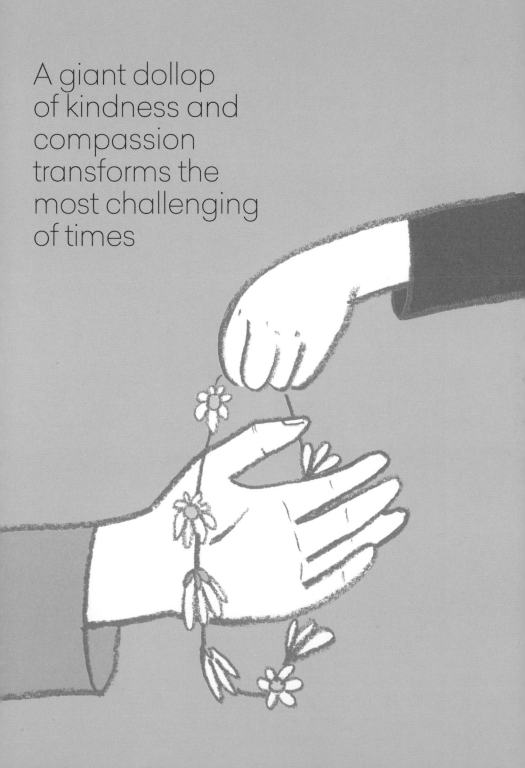

you would your best friend". If it's not right for your best buddy, it's not right for you either. Gently reframe what you've said and feel the difference it makes. There truly is no glory in tearing yourself down. For adults and older children, another way to cultivate self-compassion is to look at a photo of their younger self and ask, "Would it be ok to talk unkindly to this little person?" There is no difference between what was right for you then and what is right for you, and any human being, now.

» **Curiosity and awe.** The desire to learn, inquisitiveness and being on the lookout for awe are all wonderful mood boosters. The simple words "I wonder" break us free from habit and rigidity and remind us that it's ok to be a beginner. Rather than rushing in to "fix" or deliver the answers, encouraging your children to source their own solutions and strategies is a good practice. The simple question "What could you do differently next time?" can be an effective way to stimulate resourcefulness and self-reliance. Curiosity can also promote greater empathy and connection. Rather than leaping to single conclusions, ask your child to get curious about how others might be feeling and generate lots of possible explanations for behaviour.

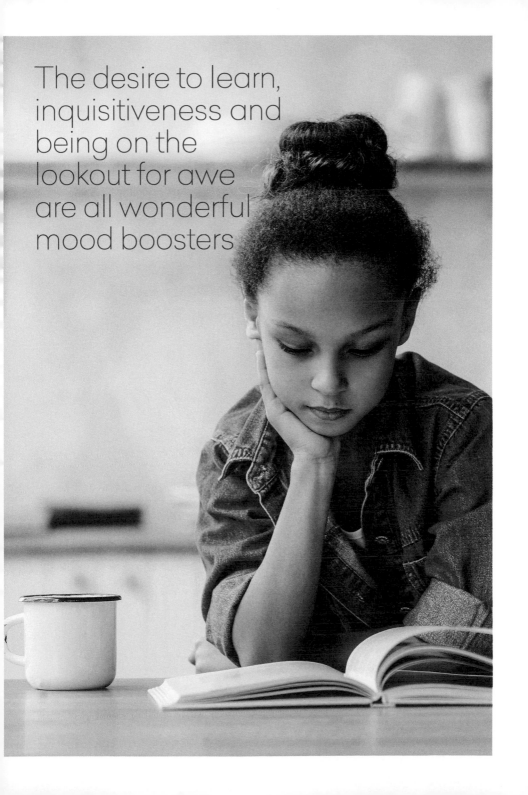

The desire to learn, inquisitiveness and being on the lookout for awe are all wonderful mood boosters

» **Appreciation and gratitude.** And the greatest mood alchemists for last. Appreciation is the skill of noticing what is good in our lives and gratitude is the quality of thankfulness for our blessings and the opportunities to grow, the silver lining to our struggles. What are the ways that you can imbed these qualities into your family life, drawing you deeply together?

» Bring back grace at the dinner table or, when the mood is right, have a celebratory gratitude dinner where you give voice to the good things in your life.

» Get skilled in the art of looking someone in the eye and saying thank you.

» Write a letter of thanks, stating what the kindness was and how it has enriched your life.

» Let people know how much you appreciate their efforts and friendship.

» Encourage an attitude of appreciation for the physical body and a feeling of thankfulness for the amazing things it allows you to do rather than being hung up on its form.

» Make a "tree of gratitude" in your home, reflecting on your collective blessings and hang it somewhere you'll see regularly.

» Quit comparing yourself to those you perceive to have more – notice those who have less and feel thankful (social media has a lot to blame here).

» At school pick-up, ask your child one thing they were grateful for in their day and offer something from your day too.

» At the end of the day, write in your Self-Care Journal three things that went well and why they happened. On days when this is a tough exercise, read through some of your older gratitude entries. Feel how this paves the way for a more peaceful night's sleep.

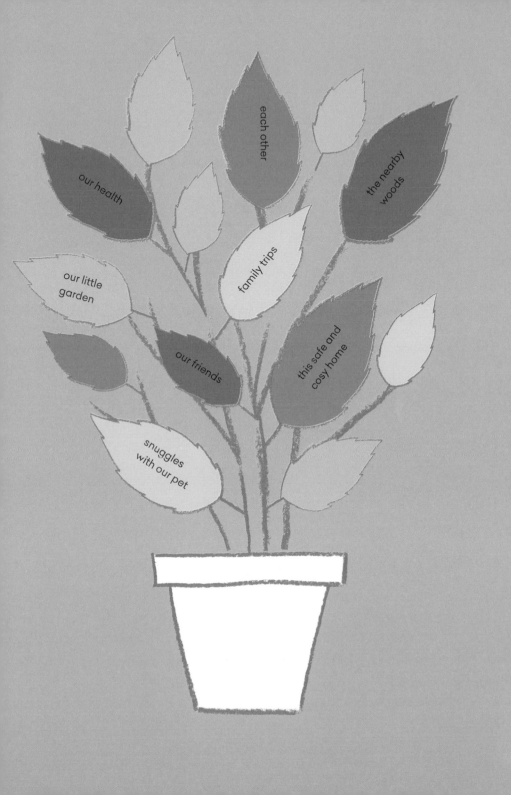

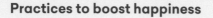
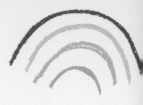

Practices to boost happiness

Play

Build a library of games, puzzles, cards and dress-ups. Engage in imaginative role play. Have options that children can play on their own or with others.

Art and creativity

The sky is the limit here. Write a song or poem. Make a book. Paint, draw or colour in. Get the chalk out on the garden path or paint on it with water. Make a sculpture from clay or build a creation from the contents of the recycling container. Try some sand art, make a mosaic or get creative with finger knitting or sewing. Bake a cake or make some freshly squeezed orange juice – zesty fun!

Display your family values

Create a poster with a mantra or statement of what's important to you. One of our favourites: "*I matter, other people matter, everyone matters.*"

Move your body

Any movement has a potential anti-depressant effect and a tall, upright posture creates a more buoyant mood. For some lightheartedness, try the yoga poses on pages 106–7.

Make a smile

Even if you don't feel it initially – the brain can't tell the difference. Fake a smile and it will help lift your mood. Even better, find a buddy, sit and look into each other's eyes and smile. Feel how this builds a sense of connection and mutual care and, most probably, laughter.

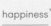

Build a happiness library

Read or watch something funny, make a joke book, or watch a YouTube puppy video. *George of the Jungle* is one of our go-to happy films.

Sing or listen to music

We've had many an impromptu dance party with our little karaoke machine and microphone. Music can also transform times that are often fraught with stress, such as car journeys, getting ready for school or preparing for bedtime.

Shift the collective mood by using scent

My kids love my room sprays, scented candles and pillow spray as much as I do.

Meditate

You can close your eyes and feel your breathing, repeat a mantra or simply notice around you anything you find beautiful or uplifting, such as nature's splendour, interesting buildings, sounds, people or colours you love.

Visualize your "Best Day Ever"

No limits here, close your eyes and fill your whole day with the best food, the best people, the best places and the best activities you can possibly imagine.

Make a "memory bank"

Use your Self-Care Journal to record happy memories and photos. Write down what happened, why it happened (there is no right or wrong here but it'll boost your mood pondering it) and get as descriptive as you can about how it made you feel in terms of thoughts, emotions and sensations. Reading these entries back later will help you re-experience the pleasure.

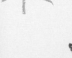

happiness

YOGA POSES TO LIFT YOUR MOOD

DOWNWARD DOG "ON A TREE"

Purpose: this one always makes us giggle.

From all fours, as you breathe in, lift your hips up and your knees off the floor. As you breathe out, let your head hang freely and bring your heels toward the floor, creating an upside down "V" shape. Lift one leg up high, bending the knee and hang out here for a few breaths before trying the other leg.

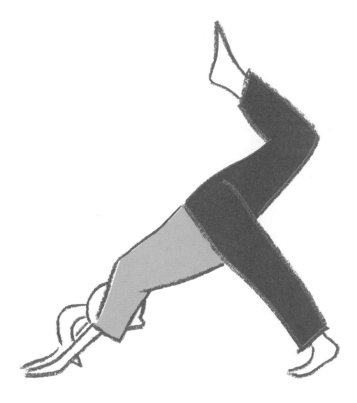

COBRA POSE

Purpose: opens the heart and strengthens the back.

Lie down on your tummy with your palms placed by your chest. As you breathe out, lift your chest, head and neck skyward, keeping your arms bent and your shoulders away from your ears. Feel this stretch the front of your body. Hissing optional.

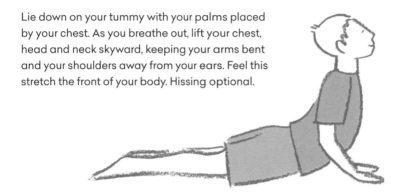

STANDING TWIST

Purpose: to feel light and free.

Stand with your feet shoulder-width apart, swing both of your arms around to the right-hand side of your body, turning in the same direction, then repeat to the other side. Let your arms be floppy and totally relaxed. Twist at least six times to each side, feeling the joyfulness of this movement.

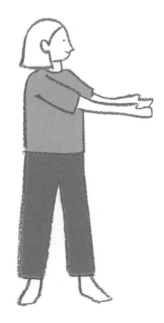

When I feel happy I will...

» This one is super simple...when I feel happy I will savour it! I will give the experience my full attention, amplifying it with my mind. I will feel it with all my senses. I deserve to feel happy, everyone does.

» If I can, I might share it with people around me so we can all enjoy it.

» I might choose to draw it or write about what happened in my Self-Care Journal, building my "memory bank" of happy moments.

When I feel sad I will...

» Remind myself that this feeling will pass and that it's ok to feel sad. I'll ask myself what my sadness is telling me. Do I need to do anything? Sometimes there's nothing to be done.

» I might choose to sit with the feeling, noticing where it is in my body, or I might imagine it as a colour or type of weather. I'll notice how it changes with time too.

» I can talk about it with someone I trust or I can write down or draw on a piece of paper what is bothering me. I can pop it in my Worry Box (see page 129) and let it go.

» I can ask for help from my family, a friend or a teacher.

» If I choose, I can dip into my Happiness Treasure Box and look for an activity that appeals to me. I give myself permission to feel happy when the time is right.

» I can try some yoga poses such as Ladybird (page 68) or Stand Tall Like a Mountain (page 46) or I could just find a safe place, lie down and do some balloon belly breathing (see page 66).

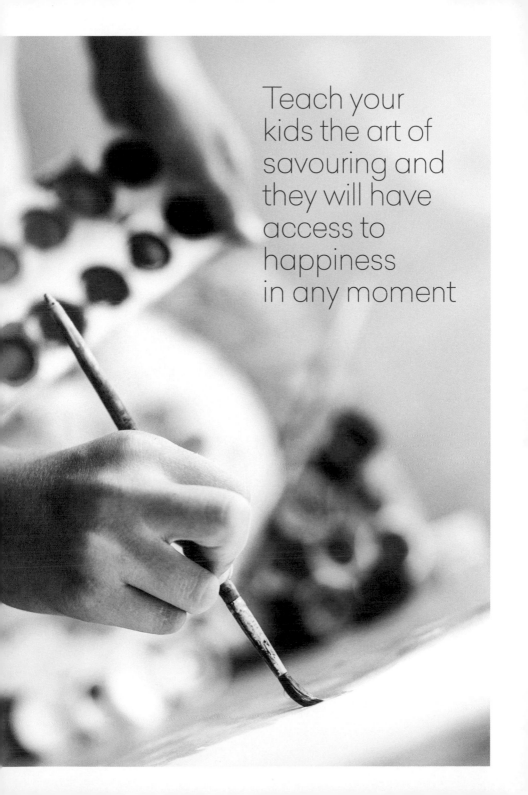

Teach your
kids the art of
savouring and
they will have
access to
happiness
in any moment

FIVE

EAT & MOVE

Healthy nutrition, hydration and daily movement are essential for feeling good and there are lots of ways that we can cultivate collective healthy habits. I spent a decade working as a personal trainer so I have lots of inspiration to share that will get you and your family moving. I'm not a nutritionist so my focus in this chapter is on the psychology of healthy lifestyle change. We'll explore the strategies and tools that promote healthy eating and exercise, maximizing the collective nourishment and enjoyment gleaned from both. It's about empowering your kids with the "WHY" (see page 112), active role-modelling, planning, encouraging ownership, and most importantly, seeking a sense of fun.

HEALTHY EATING

The mantra for sustainable healthy eating is: *"Make good choices most of the time"*. The fundamental message we try to communicate to our kids is that we need to fill up on whole, fresh foods. We conceptualize "junk" food (sugary desserts, chocolate, salty snacks, cookies and cakes) as a treat to be savoured, not as "food" for sustenance. They know they must fill up to fuel their health first and treats may come afterward. And the mantra when it comes to treats is: *"If I'm going to indulge, then I'm going to savour it"*. Relish your dessert or pizza and movie night with every fibre of your body!

Empowering your kids with the knowledge of what different types of foods do and why they need them can encourage them to get on board with better nutritional choices. Knowing the "WHY" of healthy eating itself motivates your kids intrinsically rather than relying on your constant bleating. You don't have to get elaborate with your explanations, any benefit that is related to something personally motivating for your kids is more galvanizing than "because it's good for you". On the following page are some benefits to inspire you.

THE WHY OF HEALTHY EATING

Feed your brain. We need good nutrition to be able to think straight. It is essential for concentration, focus, attention and your memory. Eating healthy food will boost your creativity and resourcefulness too. You also need to eat well so you can sleep and switch off.

Nourish your mood. Want to feel happy, calm, optimistic, patient, compassionate, kind, or enjoy a sense of humour? Then eat healthy, life-giving foods and drink water at regular intervals.

Fuel your body. Choose foods that give you energy to last the day, for physical activity, cellular growth and renewal, strength, stamina, pep and vigour!

HEALTHY HYDRATION

Good hydration is essential for healthy functioning. According to the British Nutrition Foundation, the amount of fluid a child needs depends on a few factors including their age, the weather and amount of physical activity, but generally they should aim to drink about 6–8 glasses of water a day. Serving sizes vary depending on age – younger children need relatively small servings (e.g. 120–150ml/4–5fl oz) and older children need larger servings (e.g. 250–300ml/8–10fl oz)[9]. It's not necessarily easy getting fluids into kids and we've resorted to every type of cup/bottle/straw combination possible because novelty really helped fluid intake. Fizzy drinks are firmly off the radar in our household because, tooth decay aside, self-regulation of emotion and behaviour becomes *impossible* for little ones in the throes of the sugar/colouring highs.

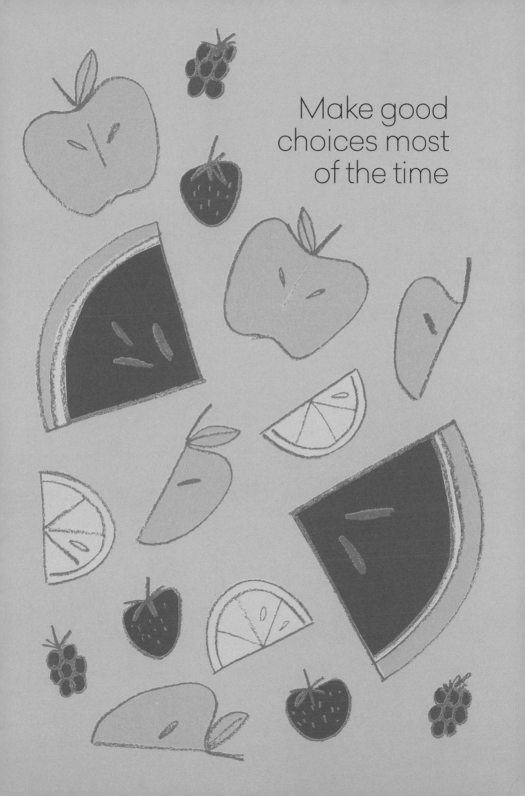

Make good
choices most
of the time

EMOTIONAL HEALTH AND MEALTIMES

Many parents are driven around the bend by their children's eating, and this is what I have learned along the way: it's not just what your children are ingesting that has an impact on their well-being, it's also the environment in which they eat. I think this helps to temper our expectations of ourselves and our kids, and "ideal" healthy eating goals need to be kept in balance with our ability to remain a calm, safe place at mealtimes. When I became a parent, my goal was to make sure my children had three life-giving meals, plus snacks, every day. Very soon, and with repeated learning, I came to change that goal to make sure they've had enough to keep them *alive*...
I can't MAKE them eat anything! It is better for collective well-being to make peace with your children eating a banana, toast or porridge for dinner than eating a tiny portion of the "ideal" meal under duress. The banana will keep them alive, it's ok and you can all stay friends in the process!

While we all know that a colourful diet is ideal, getting fruit and vegetables into our kids can prove challenging... Make peace with what they'll happily eat for now. It will change. Sneak in what you can in your cooked dishes and fresh smoothies. Keep trying different foods. Try the "smell, lick, tiny bite" approach and praise them for each mini trial for the true accomplishment that it is. Work with what you've got and avoid traumatizing yourself and your kids with rigid ideals.

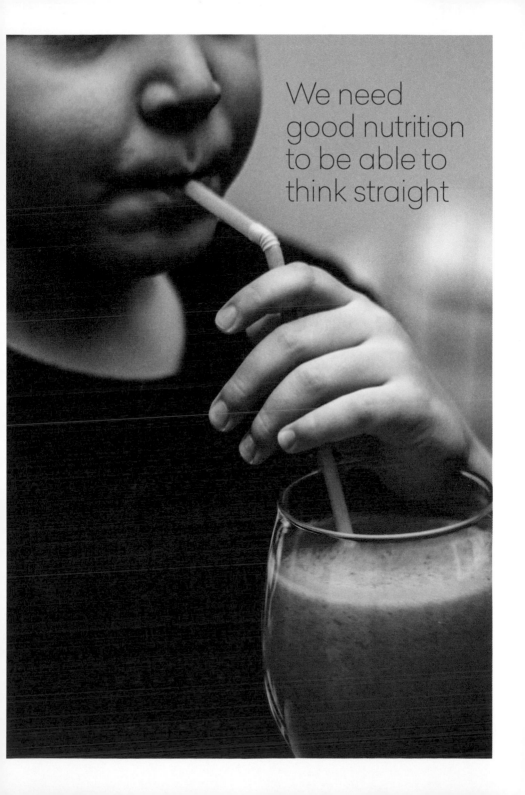

We need
good nutrition
to be able to
think straight

A note on gut health and the mind

There is a wealth of new research and resources available on gut health, highlighting the link between the human microbiome and mood[10]. As a psychologist, I am passionate about raising awareness of the interconnection between gut health and mental health. I often have clients calling in the midst or aftermath of physical illness, especially stomach bugs and viruses, complaining of acute symptoms of anxiety and depression. If you're unwell, don't be surprised if your mood is low or your thinking is sticky. I find this is really useful to know, to communicate with your kids, helping them remember there is a reason for it and it is likely to pass. We promote a healthy functioning gut by exercising regularly, getting adequate sleep, encouraging relaxation, creating a healthy environment (do ditch the antibacterial hand sanitizer though) and through our diet. Boost gut health with your nutrition by eating a wide range of plant-based foods, getting plenty of fibre, avoiding sugar and highly processed foods, and consuming probiotic foods such as live yogurt, some cheeses and fermented foods which can encourage microbes to grow. This becomes even more crucial after a bout of antibiotics which kill "good" bacteria as well as "bad".

PRACTICAL TIPS TO BOOST HEALTHY CHOICES & HAPPY, HARMONIOUS EATING

PLAN AND ORGANIZE

This is the absolute bottom line. If healthy food isn't readily available in the house, in "hanger" we all turn to convenience or junk food. Sit down with your family and create a meal plan for the coming week. Base your grocery shopping on what you'll need and you'll collectively eat better and reduce waste. Prepare meals in batches so on busy evenings you have some healthy options at fingertips' reach. The easiest thing has to be healthy, so we keep the house stocked with things such as yogurt, edamame beans, berries, avocados, bananas, carrots that I cut for the kids so they can just dive in, wholemeal pitta in the freezer which is fab when freshly toasted with hummus, nuts and seeds. Treats are kept out of eye view and out of reach for those who can't resist temptation. Make a list of the nourishing foods that you enjoy as a family and make sure these are routinely on the shopping list.

EAT REGULAR LIFE-GIVING MEALS AND RESPECT HUNGER

To nourish mood and mental clarity it is especially important that we eat at regular intervals. We literally need to feed the brain so we can make good decisions including on what we consume. Encourage your children to get to know and respect their hunger. Eat something nutritious when you are hungry and stop eating when you are full. For kids with small appetites it might be useful to eat first and then drink. Another approach that helps is to keep portion sizes small on the plate. I dish up what I hope they'll eat at a minimum – if they want more they can have more. A plate piled high with food can be overwhelming. It pays to be mindful of how tiny their little tummies are too! It doesn't take much to feel full so allow them to respect their body's feeling of fullness. Ask if there's space for a treat, however, for a more honest answer...

eat & move

PREPARE YOUR MEALS TOGETHER

Cooking with your kids is a wonderful mindfulness exercise – park any worries while you prepare and enjoy a life-giving meal together. Cooking with children is bonding and builds their skills which in turn boosts their self-esteem. Explain your techniques and why you're doing what you're doing. Share with them your precious family recipes – this creates a sense of lineage and keeps that connection alive. My daughter likes to record these in her Self-Care Journal and I hope she will keep revisiting them as she grows up. Are there dishes your children want to learn how to cook? This can encourage tricky eaters to try new things. I find that meals my children have helped prepare are devoured with far greater interest and relish.

MAKE MEAL TIMES A RITUAL OF COMING TOGETHER

Get your children involved in setting the table, bringing over dishes and say grace or a word of gratitude together. Leave books, toys and phones elsewhere and set the intention to share the experience of eating. Find out what's happened in each other's day, boosting your feeling of connection. Meal times provide us with another ideal opportunity to practise mindfulness – savouring the colours of your food, the aromas, the sensations, the taste and texture of food in the mouth and sharing what you're finding pleasurable. I eat dinner with my children, a small symbolic portion of whatever they are having, and also eat later with my husband when he gets home. If you choose to do this too, be sensible with portion sizes and don't feel you have to finish what's left on your children's plates. If you are constantly throwing food away, take a look at the volume you are preparing and make some adjustments. Clearing away gives another opportunity for sharing responsibilities and your children might love the mindfulness of washing up too.

"HELP YOURSELF" AND ENCOURAGE CHOICE

Some of the most pleasurable meal times have come in the form of a sharing plate or feast where we can all help ourselves and choose what we'd like to eat. The social aspect to this often encourages dabbling in different foods. Kids enjoy feeling responsible and grown up. It's ok to provide a boundary to the choices – it's not "Would you like any vegetables?", it is "Which ones would you like?"

MAKE IT PRETTY AND FUN

A vase of flowers, tablecloths, place mats, plates, cups and cutlery you all enjoy can make a genuine difference to meal times.

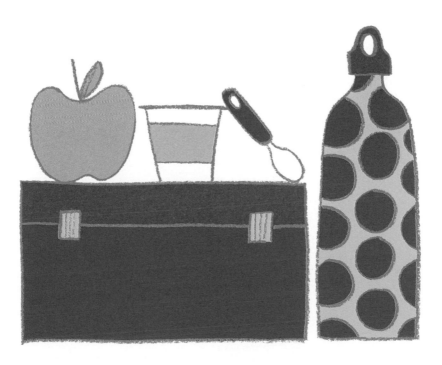

HEALTHY MOVEMENT

It's not just sport or "exercise", any movement can have far-reaching benefits for individual and collective health and well-being. Don't just encourage your kids to move, move with them. They literally follow your lead. There are so many ways to boost physical movement in your day. Take a look at your schedule and identify ways that you can get a little more activity into your week, whether it is walking a little further, getting out into the garden or trying some yoga at home together. Plan it in your week and make appointments in the calendar to give it the priority it deserves. Talk to your kids about the benefits of movement and draw their attention to how much better they feel after moving their bodies, building their self-care toolkit. If the movement you're choosing isn't intrinsically enjoyable, do something else. It doesn't need to be unappealing or painful or even feel like exertion for it to have wide-reaching health benefits. The keys to sustainable healthy movement are:

» Commitment

» Prioritizing

» Planning

» Engaging in enjoyable pursuits

Need more convincing? There'll be something appealing when you look at the benefits:

THE WHY OF HEALTHY MOVEMENT

Move for your MIND. It's not just about shaping your physical body, the mantra is *"Move for mental health"*. Movement lifts your mood and boosts your creativity, problem-solving, focus, attention and memory. Feel blue, bored, stuck in your thoughts or caught in procrastination? Move your body and feel the shift of energy this creates. Try a Downward Dog (see page 69) and you might literally see things from a different perspective.

Move for your BODY. We're all aware of the benefits of movement in building strength, coordination, suppleness and growth, but recognize too that movement fuels an appreciation for your physical capacity and what it allows you to do[11]. Encourage your kids to appreciate function over form. From that place of gratitude for your body grows a feeling of empowerment and a more positive body image[12].

Move for your HEART. And I'm not talking about the cardiovascular system here – move to nurture friendships and build connection. Team sports provide a fabulous feeling of belonging, and moving with your loved ones can be a life-giving way to share time and make memories together. Your shared movement goals can also bring you together and propel you on to greater achievements.

Aim for 30 minutes a day and remember that *any* movement counts. Movement has a cumulative effect so it needn't be an unbroken stretch of 30 minutes. Five minutes here and there will have the same health benefits. Variety will help boost motivation and keep your body responding and a mix of aerobic exercise, resistance-based work and stretching is preferable. No need to a join a gym (unless you want to!) – all you need is your own body and some inspiration. Get to know yourself, the genuine barriers and the excuses that crop up. Proactively generate some primer statements to help you make the commitment to regular exercise. Think along the lines of "If I am feeling tired, then I will try some yoga stretches" or "If it's raining and netball is cancelled, then I will pop on some music and do some lunges, squats and tummy curls inside."

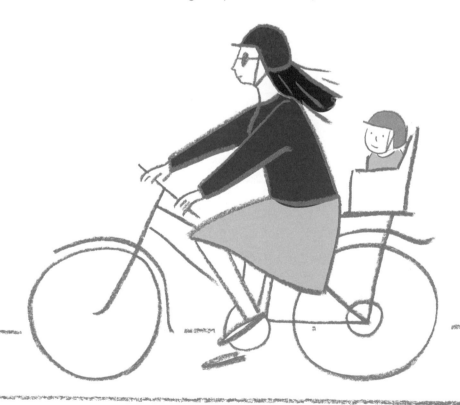

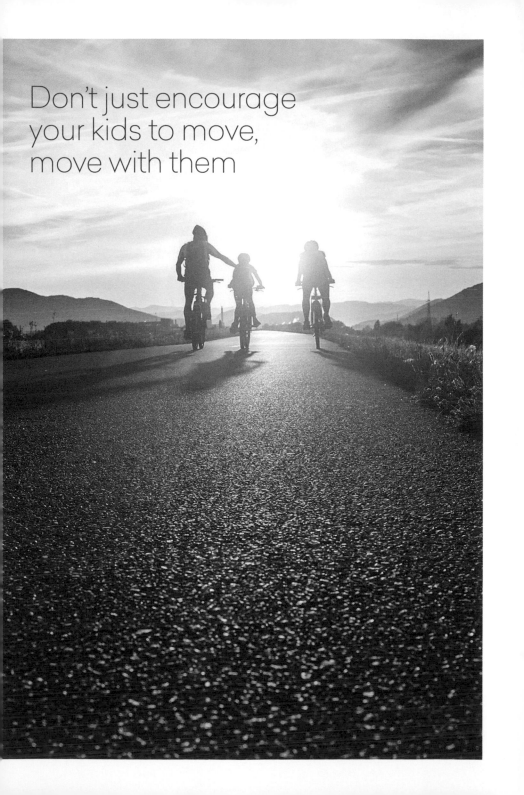

Don't just encourage
your kids to move,
move with them

Practices to get moving

Brainstorm with your family all the different ways that you can move and jot them down on your "Eat and Move" section of the Vitality Wheel. Turn to it whenever you need a collective boost or there's a window to move your body! Here are some ideas:

Dance

Pop on some tunes or music videos and move. Boogie while you're doing chores.

Yoga

There is some in every chapter, catering for all moods and energy levels.

Garden

Mow, do some weeding, watering, planting or try a handstand on the soft grass.

Tidy up

Vacuuming, dusting, cleaning the windows, folding and putting away the laundry all count.

Walk or jog

Just go around the block or take a longer nature walk. Seek out some hills, steps or throw in some walking lunges, bench dips or press ups. If you're after an excuse to get a dog, look no further.

Play games

Try old-fashioned favourites such as skipping, hopscotch and Twister, or introduce a bit of technology and use your Wii Fit.

Kick a ball

Get outside to the nearest green space and have an impromptu kickaround, or a quick game of frisbee.

Cycle, scoot or walk places to which you might ordinarily drive

Try these new, more active modes of transport to places rather than using the car.

Visit a local farm or zoo

Better still, take out a family membership and use it as an opportunity to get out and about together regularly.

Water play

On hot days get out the sprinkler or go to a local pool and have a splash about together.

Get adventurous

Try ice skating, indoor ski slopes, kayaking, trampolining or rock climbing.

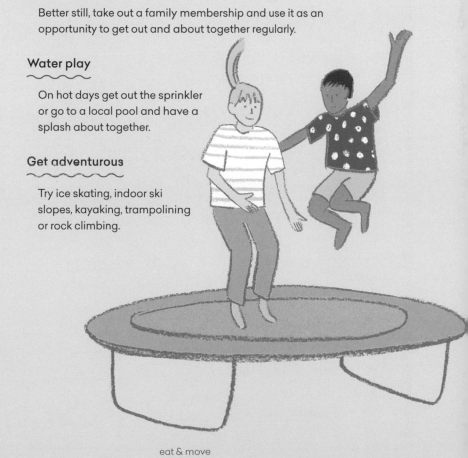

YOGA TO GET YOU MOVING

HORSE POSE TO STAR BALANCE

Purpose: to get the heart rate going and strengthen your whole body.

Start with your feet one-and-a-half times shoulder-width apart and toes pointing out to 45 degrees. Sink into a squat with your hands together at your heart. Stand up and bring your weight onto your right foot and lift your left leg up, tipping over into a star shape and hover. Come back into the squat and repeat the Star Balance to the other side. Repeat six times each side.

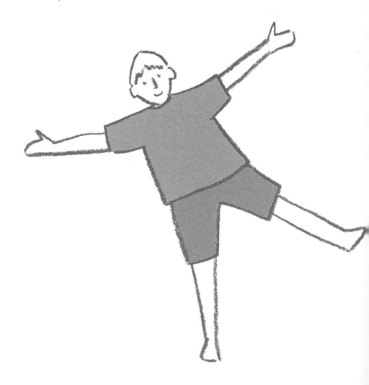

KNEELING SUPERMAN

Purpose: to strengthen the back of your body.

Begin on all fours with your spine in "neutral",
ensuring there is no sagging of your back and
abdomen throughout this sequence. Inhale:
reach your right arm out forward, thumb pointing
upward and your left leg out behind you, with the
back heel flexed. Exhale: come back to all fours,
keeping your hips and your shoulders level. Inhale:
extend your left arm and right leg out. Exhale:
return to all fours. Feel the strength and support
of your core muscles and enjoy the feeling of
extending your spine. Repeat 6–10
times each side.

BRIDGE POSE

Purpose: to stretch your tummy and fire up
your legs.

On your back with your knees bent, feet on the
floor, breathe in and lift your arms over to the
floor above your head. Breathe out, lift your hips
skyward and bring your arms back down by your
sides. Breathe in: arms up and hips down. Breathe
out: hips up, arms down. Repeat ten times.

When I feel anxious I will...

» **Remind myself** that anxious thoughts and feelings are normal. I can just let it be. I won't give myself a hard time and get worried about feeling worried.

» **Use a mantra:** *"This is just a thought or a feeling. It will pass. It won't be like this forever"*.

» **Scan my body** and soften any physical tension I find – especially my face, eyes, jaw, shoulders and chest.

» **Use my posture to feel better.** Stand tall with an open heart, feel the length of my spine, the strength of my legs and the support of the earth beneath me.

» **Breathe.** Try balloon belly breathing (see page 66) and make my exhalations long and smooth.

» **Move.** A regular yoga practice will help manage a tendency to feel anxious in as little as five minutes a day. To help in anxious times, turn to Stand Tall Like a Mountain (page 46), Ladybird pose (page 68), or Standing Twist (page 107). A simple walk in nature can calm and ground me too.

» **Distract myself.** Use my Mindfulness Jar (see page 30) or anchor my mind on something uplifting like my Self-Care Journal, music I love or something beautiful or funny.

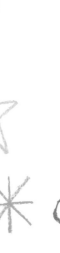
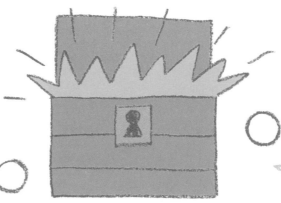

» **Reframe.** Ask myself, "Is this concern real, can I do anything about it?", "Will this matter in a year?" or "What am I learning here?"

» **Eat and hydrate.** Is my anxiety a function of being hungry or dehydrated? Have a life-giving snack and a glass of water.

» **Touch.** Seek out a hug or sit and stroke a pet. Cuddly toys have their place too.

» **Express it.** I can write down my worries and enjoy tossing them away or put them in a "Worry Box" for safe keeping, so I can then let them go. Give voice to my worries with a parent. Just saying them out loud can clarify what's real and what's not. Write myself a letter as if penned to a friend, talking about my worry. If worry is persistent, give myself a specific time to worry. When anxious thoughts pop up outside of that time, I'll remind myself it's not time for that now.

» **Be kind.** Doing something nice for someone else can take me out of my own head and being of service to other people is a great way to shift my mood. I'll be kind and gentle to me too.

SIX

CONNECT

Connection feeds the individual soul and fuels the heart of the family. Healthy, positive relationships form a cornerstone of well-being and many would say that belonging and relationships are what life is all about. Humans have a basic, evolutionary need to belong, to love and feel loved. It is in relationship with others that our rough edges are smoothed away, family life providing insight for each member on what's ok and how to make the most of our strengths. This spoke of the Vitality Wheel explores the simple skills and habits that draw families together, deepening bonds and our ability to relate to one another, providing our kids with a secure foundation from which to explore the world.

WHAT IS CONNECTION?

Connection is created when we bring the skills of mindfulness and compassion to our interactions with other people. It is about feeling in tune with another person, a sense of being in this moment together. It comes about by the communication of either mutual care, experience or interest. It can be as simple as eye contact and a nod to greet a passerby, showing that "you're in it together". It can be found in lighthearted conversation with the person next to you at the lunch table or the person serving you at a checkout. With those you love, it can be tuning in to hear about the goings on of their day, a kind gesture, the resting of a hand on a shoulder, or an embrace. Connection feels like you've plugged into an energy source, filling life with purpose and zest, making it a potent means of nourishment.

BUILDING CONNECTION WITHIN THE FAMILY

What feeds a relationship and the health of the family unit? Currency, time to be together, the quality of our communication, shared experience and memory-making all keep a family unit feeling cohesive and connected. Let's explore each in greater depth:

CURRENCY

This is about being up to date with each other, knowing what's going on in each other's lives and communicating presence. Ask questions about what's coming up so you can check in that evening. I appreciate this is difficult during our children's monosyllabic phases, but persevere. Currency also comes in sharing your interests, creating a feeling of being known and understood, so asking your children what they found interesting in their day can be a good starting point. You can wrap someone up in love whether you are physically present or not. My mother stays current by writing letters and emailing funny videos to the kids. We keep our connection lively by sending her images of what we're up to. None of these things takes long but the dividends are tangible.

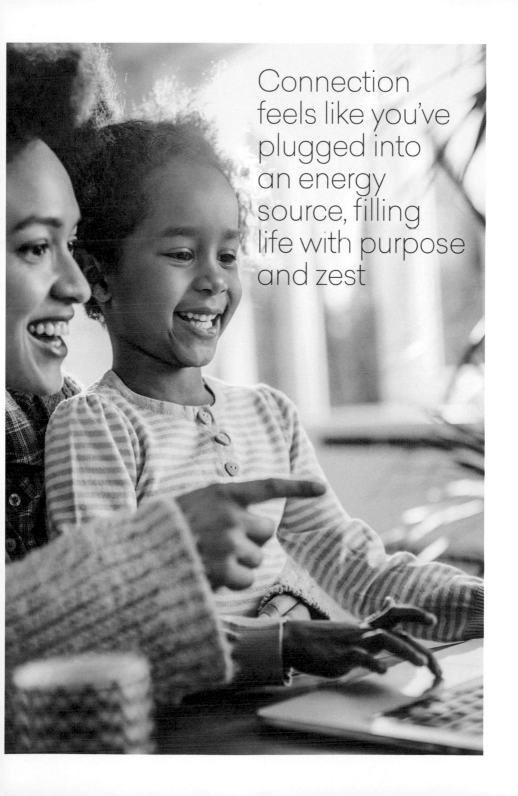

Connection feels like you've plugged into an energy source, filling life with purpose and zest

MAKE TIME TO BE TOGETHER

Quality time can be engaging in shared activities or just sharing space. If there are things you enjoy doing together, savour those experiences. Sometimes it's enough just to be in the same room together, enjoying individual pursuits. The connection comes in noticing and appreciating that you are all together.

Creating a ritual at the school gate or a coming together at the end of the day keeps families feeling bonded. How you reconnect is totally up to you – it could be sharing a meal, sitting down to process your day or enjoying a relax in front of the tv together. You can imbue many different activities with the intention to reconnect. Are there particular things that you like to do as a family to mark coming together on the weekend? We love piling into bed and having a family snuggle before we embark on the various sporting and social commitments on weekend mornings. Cooking together and enjoying nature are other rituals of connection.

COMMUNICATION

The family unit is kept healthy by prioritizing time to give voice to thoughts, feelings and ideas, welcoming the input of others by inviting comment and feedback. Connection is boosted by active listening where you show genuine interest in what's being said with eye contact, nodding, asking questions, and paraphrasing to confirm that you've understood correctly. It's not just the time to talk, it is how you talk to each other. Especially for little ones, getting down to their eye level will help you gain their attention and will make you feel a safer place than if you are towering over them. If you find it hard to get your kids' attention I recommend the Ricky Gervais YouTube video with his cat Colin[13]... It's worth a watch, trust me. If my kids aren't responding to their names, I say "Colin" a few times and we can all have a giggle.

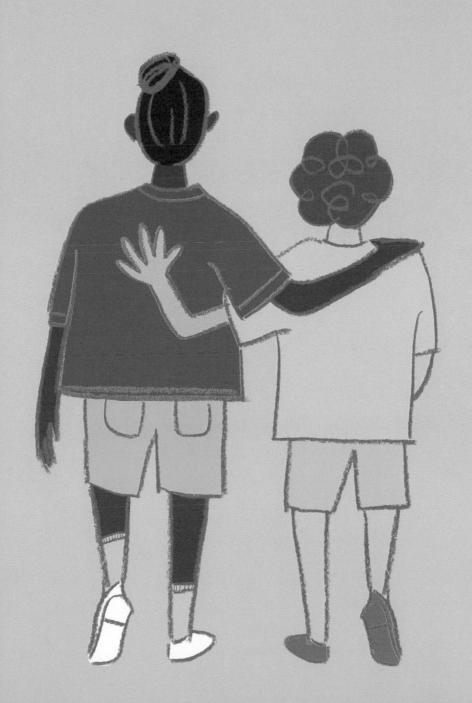

Bringing mindfulness to conversation is a wonderful practice, giving you the opportunity to step back and choose words that are most constructive. "Nonviolent communication" is the key here and, granted, this is not easy when tempers are flaring. Nonviolent communication is about addressing behaviour, rather than evoking blame, criticism or attacking the person:

"You are so unkind" becomes "What you just said or did was unkind."

"What's wrong with you?" becomes "What's the matter?"

We can also practise nonviolent communication by leading with an observation without emotional attachment and gently asking a question to find out more, such as "You haven't said much this evening. Is there something on your mind?" The ratio of positive to negative statements has an impact on the health of relationships too. Aim for a ratio of three positive remarks for every negative one, which means for parents, we need to become skilled in praising what our children are doing well, not just giving voice to what we want to change.

CREATING MEMORIES AND RELIVING THEM

Happy memories bond us together and build our feeling of shared identity. Reminiscing about them boosts the collective mood. What are some of your most poignant family memories and how can you go about creating new ones? Family outings or holidays are a wonderful way of making significant markers but, equally, they can be found in the simple things. I am grateful to my father for sharing with us his favourite songs because we stay connected with him whenever we hear them and I love that we can feel close to Nana and Grandad by sharing their love of gardening. Enjoy building your "memory bank" in your Self-Care Journal and revisiting it together.

Grief: a note on staying connected after loss

There is no right or wrong way to grieve, no timetable to grief and how people express and experience it is deeply personal. I hope that some of the soothing yoga poses in this book might be a place to start in moving through grief. In my experience, seeking ways to build a continued relationship after death has been healing for the whole family. Children are remarkably open to the idea and create their own ways to stay connected. A feeling that someone is "gone" can be utterly heartbreaking. Thinking of the person changing forms or being present in other ways can soften this blow. They're not gone, they're just here in a different way. Your connection is kept alive by thought, conversation, and engagement in meaningful activities or by visiting significant places. Grandpa is no longer here in bodily form but he is conjured every time we hear ABBA. He comes to visit us in the garden in the shape of birds and butterflies. He has visited me as a kingfisher on several poignant moments – the day of his funeral and the morning my son started nursery.

BOOSTING CONNECTION OUTSIDE THE FAMILY UNIT: WHO'S ON YOUR TEAM?

In addition to our family, we need our friends to support us, cheer us on and to celebrate the good times. It is helpful to acknowledge that connection comes in many different forms and the purpose of those relationships can vary. Having a broad set of friendships on which to draw is a wonderful thing and the concept that's useful here is thinking about who's on your team.

Think about all the people you hold dear in life and jot them down or get creative and make some kind of diagram. There might be extended family, people from school/work, teachers, buddies from sport or other activities, coaches or neighbours. Jot down next to each name the kind of activities you enjoy doing with them or maybe their strengths. You will notice that different people have different strengths and how you enjoy time with them varies. Some friends provide a kind ear, others you just want to play sports with, and that's ok. Get to know what each person on your team does well and enjoy that strength. Consider what you bring to the table too and make sure it's a two-way street.

Check in with your list and make sure you're staying current with the special people on your team, nourishing those relationships. Notice that friendships change with time and that some might naturally fall away as your interests or other life variables change. This is a normal part of life.

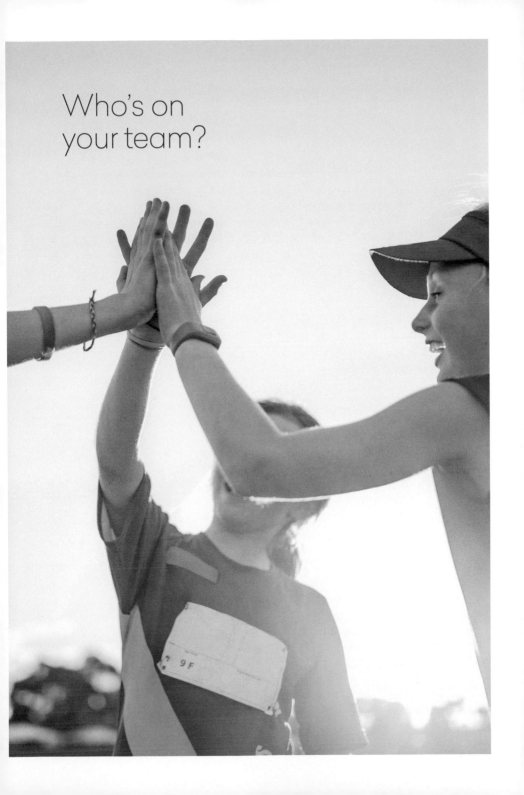

Who's on
your team?

Practices to boost connection

Reflect on what friendship or family means to you

What qualities do you value? Think about the people dear to you and write down what you appreciate about your relationship in your Self-Care Journal. Maybe it is trust, laughter, a safe place to share or mutual interests. There is no right or wrong. Expressing this appreciation with your friends and loved ones is a wonderful way to build greater closeness. It's ok to invest in the relationships that feel most nourishing and uplifting to you, the ones where you both value the same things or make the same kind of efforts. It's ok to choose who you spend your time and energy with.

Draw your family tree

Use it to share happy anecdotes about each member, bringing them to life for your kids. They enjoy seeing you and themselves in this greater context, creating a deeper sense of lineage and belonging.

Don't let your "cuddle cup" run empty

We like to think we all have a cup that gets filled with cuddles. When we're feeling low we let each other know we need refilling. Kids enjoy filling up with cuddles without feeling needy for asking. A mention of the cuddle cup at the right moment can circumvent undesirable behaviour – theirs and mine!

Share music together

Research has found that people who shared musical experiences with their parents during childhood report better-quality relationships with them as they enter early adulthood[14]. Foster a feeling of synchronization and closeness by playing or listening to music together or taking your children to live events such as concerts. Keeping musical tastes in synch is another way to build common bonds.

Mantras

Repeating certain phrases can help us feel more in tune with other people or promote the kind of behaviour that boosts relationships. Try using *"Kind hands and kind words"*, or phrases such as *"I am cared for"*, *"I'm not alone"* or *"Things can get better"*. *"Hurt people, hurt people"* helps us be more patient, empathetic and make kinder attributions to the actions of others.

Meditation

Loving kindness meditation can be powerful. This is where you extend a feeling of care to yourself or other people. Start with someone you feel close to: sit quietly imagining them and repeat the words: "May they be peaceful. May they be safe. May they be happy". With practice, we can learn to extend the same feelings toward someone we are in conflict with, or someone we don't feel a natural affinity with. This not only boosts connection but a feeling of inner calm.

Let them know!

Make a friendship bracelet, write a love letter or a poem, pop a note in their lunchbox or – this is one of my favourite rituals – draw a smiley face, a few of their strengths or a happy phrase on your child's sandwich bag. It is so easy to communicate care.

YOGA POSES TO BOOST CONNECTION

HANDSTAND

Purpose: to get you laughing.

If you are feeling up for a challenge (have your playful hat on), try kicking up into a Handstand against a wall. Start with your hands shoulder-width apart at the base of a wall. Carefully kick one leg up or bunny hop both legs up to the wall behind you. This may take quite a lot of courage and practice to actually "get up". Have fun playing with it. Feel how exhilarating this is even if you don't quite make it! For kids and braver adults, try it outside unaided. Another option for kids is the Assisted Handstand. Have them stand facing you, placing their hands on your feet. Bend your knees, ask them to carefully lift up one leg, take hold and hoist them up into a Handstand, holding their ankles. Always come down into a Ladybird Pose (see page 68) after trying Handstands – if you pop up to standing you are likely to feel lightheaded.

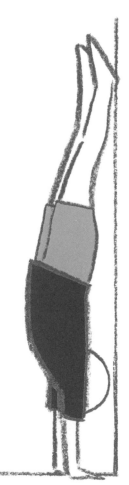

LYING DOWN KNEE HUGS

Purpose: to let go.

Lying on your back with your arms down by your sides and your legs out long, breathe in and stretch your arms above your head. As you breathe out, hug your right knee to your chest. Breathe in and lower your leg back down and reach your arms overhead. Breathe out and hug your left knee to your chest. Repeat six times with each leg and enjoy the release for your lower back and hips, blowing away what you no longer need.

LYING DOWN BUTTERFLY

Purpose: to rest in a feeling of "we're in it together".

Bring the soles of your feet together and let your knees drop toward the floor. Bring your arms to rest overhead, one hand cradled in the other. Close your eyes. Feel your belly rise and fall with your breath. Completely soften all of your body and enjoy 5–10 breaths, longer if it feels good.

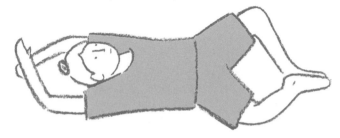

When I miss someone I will...

» Think of a happy time I spent with them.

» Remember something I really love about them – what makes them special to me?

» Look at a photo.

» Know it's ok to have a little cry.

» Fill my "cuddle cup".

» If I can, call them, and even if they're not here anymore, I can write them a letter or draw them a picture.

» Do something they loved or just remember something special to them. Maybe it's listening to a song, enjoying a dish they loved, or watching something that made them happy.

» Look for them in nature. Are they present in animals, flowers or plants?

» Think of ways I can keep a feeling of relationship alive even when we're apart or someone is no longer with us. I'll keep memories burning brightly by talking about them and happy times. I could make a memory box.

» Feel thankful for their love, say a little prayer and talk to them. My angels are always listening.

» Do something fun, maybe a little yoga pose to soothe and uplift. Try Stand Tall Like a Mountain (page 46).

When I feel lonely I will...

» Sit with the feeling a little while. Notice that I can be alone and not necessarily feel lonely. Get curious and see if there are other feelings alongside the loneliness.

» Ask "What is my loneliness prompting me to do? How would I like to feel connected with someone else?"

» Check in with who's on my team and reach out to someone who could meet my needs right now.

» Write about how I am feeling in my Self-Care Journal.

» Try some of the yoga and enjoy feeling connected with my body.

» Sit in nature's beauty or look out the window and see life at play all around me.

» Use a mantra and relax into my breathing. Try repeating: "*I am safe, I am loved, I am held*".

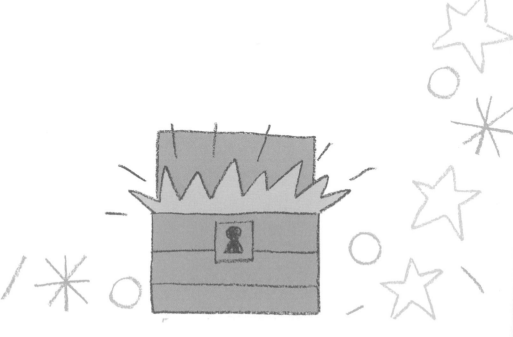

SEVEN

STRENGTHS & VALUES

There are so many different ways to shine! This chapter is all about how we communicate this message to our kids. I think every parent has had a painful experience bearing witness to real or imagined deficits at home, in the classroom or playground, our children missing out on the role they wanted on the school council or in the school play, or sporting team. We help our children enormously when we broaden their conceptualization of what it means to be "bright", introducing them to the concepts of strengths and values and helping them identify their own. When kids are aware of their strengths it can be a light-bulb moment, giving them a sense of purpose and identity. They're better placed to notice and seize their opportunities to shine, boosting self-esteem and well-being.

HOW STRENGTHS & VALUES HELP

You might be wondering, how do strengths and values relate to self-care? It is simple: using our strengths is energizing, bolstering our feelings of self-worth. Taking action in service of our values fills us with zest, allowing us to step up and make a difference. Clarity on strengths and values provides us with another superb coping strategy in our self-care toolkit. Just being aware of the concept of strengths is liberating because it teaches children that they don't have to excel at *everything*. It reminds children that their natural aptitudes will all differ, and that's ok, and that they *all* have valuable characteristics and abilities. I hope you as a parent find it equally liberating – you don't have to excel at *all* facets of parenting. Some you will rock, others will feel like a hard graft and this is all par for the course of parenthood. Being clear on our strengths boosts self-esteem and makes us feel sure of the ways that we can be a contributing member of the family, the team, the workplace or classroom. Knowing our strengths can be empowering, helping us navigate and make up for our shortfalls – for example, persistence and diligence can help you overcome weakness in mathematical ability. Just thinking about our values can be uplifting. This is why identifying and working with your strengths and values is powerful self-care, nourishing the health of the individual as well as the family as a unit.

Ask your child what "clever" means and you'll probably get a long list of abilities such as good with numbers, confident speaking, neat handwriting or reading skills, often reinforced by classroom test scores. Our children benefit when we flesh this out to include a host of other gifts involving physical capabilities, personality traits, emotions, communication, social skills and technical or creative pursuits. It's not about being better than anyone else, it is about helping them connect with the things that they naturally do well, their unique offering, and building on their opportunities to use those strengths. While there are some qualities that come more effortlessly than others, we need to highlight that there is malleability to strengths too. We can grow and develop whatever talent we choose to direct our attention to.

It is easy and very natural as parents to focus on trying to fix what our children struggle with. Rather than honing in on their weaknesses, which can be depleting and demoralizing for both of you, notice how life-giving it is to promote and expand their strengths. If you want to learn more about strengths, Professor Lea Waters is your expert. In her book *The Strength Switch*[15] she summarizes the research findings on the benefits of a strength-based approach for kids and adults alike, including:

» Greater happiness and engagement in class.

» Higher levels of academic achievement in school and college students.

» Greater happiness and better performance at work.

» Better recovery after illness.

» Higher levels of fitness and engagement in healthy lifestyle choices.

» Enhanced ability to cope with stress and adversity.

That's not to say that we give up supporting our kids when they need an extra helping hand; it's about making sure that we don't focus on weaknesses to the exclusion of the activities that make their hearts sing. It's about building awareness of both strengths and weaknesses and creating balance in how we spend our time and energy. Looking for strengths will change the lens through which you see your child, making it easier to shape behaviour and encourage self-development framed positively and constructively. You'll notice more of what they're doing well and less of what needs improvement, making for a more harmonious home environment.

interest in exploring and learning new things

diligence humility perseverance
enthusiasm loving persistence
caring loyalty gratitude
hope open minded
HONESTY FAIRNESS
BRAVERY kindness analytical
poise LEADERSHIP
forgiveness discipline
humour COMPASSION
perspective playfulness grit

WHAT ARE STRENGTHS & VALUES?

Strengths and values are inner resources, galvanizing us when life gets tough. Professor Waters defines strengths as "positive qualities that energize us, that we perform well and choose often". They are developed over time through our innate ability and dedicated effort. They are qualities recognized by others as being praiseworthy, contributing positively to the lives of others. They often come so easily that we overlook them or don't see them for the true talent they are. Values, on the other hand, are guiding principles; they are qualities that you hold dear, whether they come naturally and easily or otherwise.

HOW TO IDENTIFY STRENGTHS & VALUES

It's worth sitting down and exploring the different strengths of all your family members. It will help each member feel seen, understood and valued, all of which bring you together as a team and make for smoother interactions. On the previous page are examples from the VIA Institute on Character's character strengths but try to identify ones that resonate with you. You can just talk about interests, skills and talents with your kids, jotting down the collective observations and what's offered up organically. Once you've identified your strengths, talk about the similarities and differences between family members and reflect on how you complement each other.

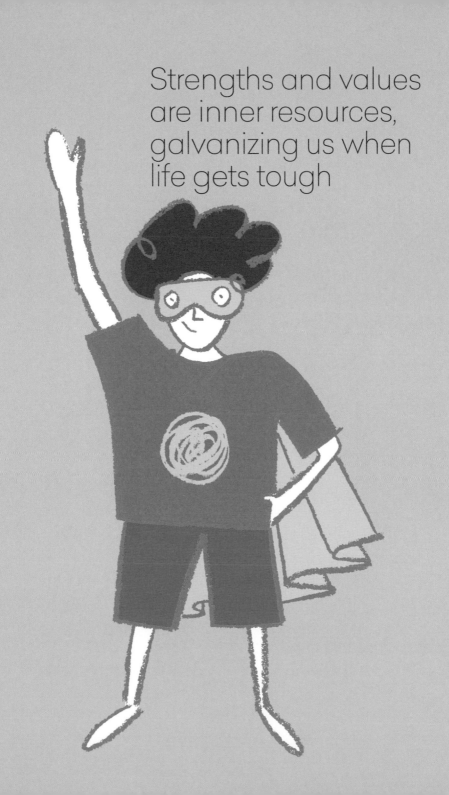

Strengths and values
are inner resources,
galvanizing us when
life gets tough

BUILDING ON STRENGTHS & VALUES

To bring strengths to life for your kids, give them concrete examples of when they've demonstrated each quality or ask them if they can think of their own examples. Keep a dialogue going about the different ways your kids can shine and when you see a strength, give voice to it. Draw their attention to when they are using their strengths and thank them for that behaviour. This will help you get the three to one ratio of positive to negative statements going! You can help your child practise their strengths by creating opportunities for them to use them or by reframing activities in a way that makes it clear how they can put their strengths into play. You can also draw their attention to how they can use their strengths to overcome challenging situations.

While we want to encourage our kids to use their strengths, it's important not to overuse them, which can be depleting or damaging to relationships. Take for example the ability to make peace among friends – just because your child is good at it doesn't mean they should be the one to compromise or bear the problem-solving responsibility all the time. Equally, if your child's strengths are honesty, humour, forgiveness or leadership, they'll need to understand when and just how much of this skill is appropriate. Any strength can be overused. Encouraging your kids to know their own strengths and those of their friends can help them better navigate the inevitable bumps in the road of friendship.

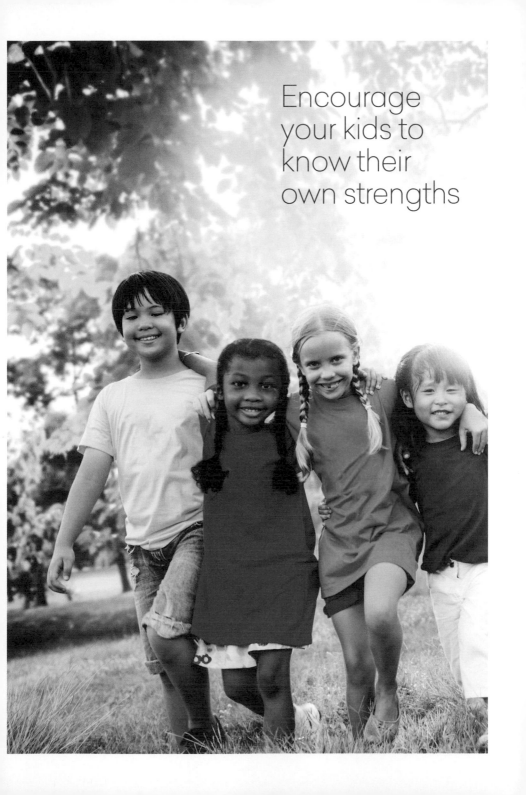

Encourage
your kids to
know their
own strengths

Practices to recognize strengths & values

Who is your hero or who inspires you and why?

What qualities do you admire? These can be real people alive right now, people from the history books or fictional characters from books, tv or film.

Map out the strengths of all your family members

Hang the map somewhere you can see it and look for ways your strengths can help around the home, making it a happy place. Show your appreciation for the strengths of others, even when they differ from yours. Getting curious about our strengths and those around us can help us understand each other better and make more charitable attributions to the behaviour of others. Because different strengths emerge developmentally at different ages it is worth revisiting this as your kids grow up, noticing how their strengths are growing and evolving.

Write a family mission statement

Be as creative as you like with colour, images, phrases, quotes or lists of qualities. Affirm what is important to you as a family. It can be as simple as "There is a lot of love in this house".

Design your personal mission statement

Jot down in your Self-Care Journal what's important to you as a person. How do you want to be in this world? What would you like to be known or remembered for? You can think about the different roles you play in life and how you'd like to be in each – for example parent, sibling, child, friend or neighbour.

In times of conflict at home

Invoke a value that you all hold dear or call on a strength that might help soothe the situation. A gentle reminder is sometimes all that's needed.

Use "I am" affirmations to channel your values

At any point in your day repeat an "I am" statement to cultivate or reinforce how you want to feel. Here are some examples we use at home: "I am calm", "I am strong", "I am capable", "I am open to learning", "I am kind". This is a wonderful practice to share with your children and if they record their affirmations in their Self-Care Journal this will continue to nourish them.

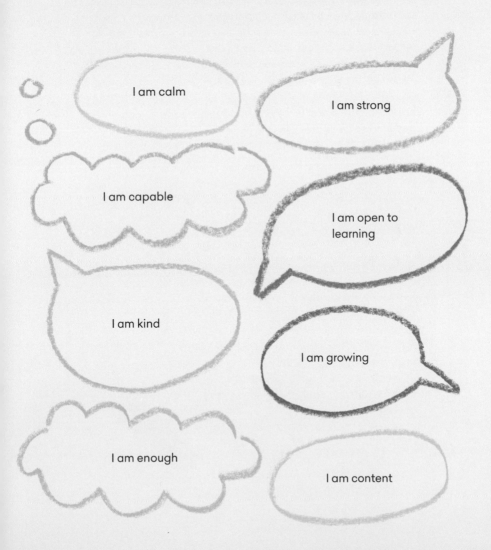

YOGA TO CONNECT YOU WITH YOUR STRENGTHS & VALUES

HORSE POSE AND MOUNTAIN BREATH

Purpose: to feel strong and energetic.

Stand with your feet one-and-a-half times shoulder-width apart and with your toes pointing out to 45 degrees. Breathe in and raise your arms out and above your head, looking up to your hands. Breathe out, bend your knees deeply, bring your arms in an arc with your fingertips touching in front of your body, gazing forward. Repeat this squatting movement slowly: lead with your breath and feel the strength of your legs and the earth beneath you. Repeat ten times.

WARRIOR POSE

Purpose: to feel strong, brave and ready.

Begin with your feet hip width apart. Think of this as standing on train tracks. Take a giant step forwards with your right foot, staying on those train tracks. Bend your right knee deeply and try to straighten your back leg – the back heel will remain off the floor. Inhale and reach your arms up and overhead to a "V" shape. Exhale and bend your elbows, lowering your arms into a "W" shape. Repeat six times before changing legs. Feel how this is uplifting and enlivening.

DANCER POSE

Purpose: for courage.

Standing, take your right heel to your right
buttock, holding the ankle with your right hand.
Without twisting, slowly take your right knee back
behind you, your left hand stretching out in front
of you and tip your chest forward, arching your
back. This takes a leap of faith! Be guided by
lightheartedness and curiosity. Hold for
5–10 breaths before changing sides.

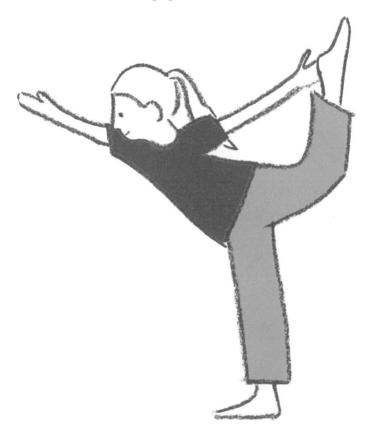

When I want to stand up for myself I will...

» Stand tall and feel the strength of my legs and the length of my spine. I can feel the earth beneath my feet, supporting me.

» Take a few deep breaths and collect myself.

» Maintain my boundaries. It is important to have boundaries and give voice to them. It's ok to want my own physical space and it's ok to want to play on my own.

» Use the words "Stop that, I don't like it".

» Call on other people for help.

» Talk about the experience later with someone I trust and come up with an action plan.

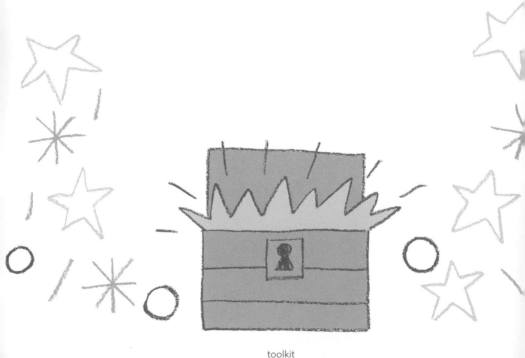

When I've made a mistake, I will...

» Breathe. It's ok, everyone makes errors...a dollop of self-compassion makes it easier to admit mistakes.

» Remember mistakes are an opportunity to grow. Pause to consider what I've learned about this scenario, this person, this relationship, or myself.

» Acknowledge that what's done is done and there's no point beating myself up over what can't be taken away.

» Step up and apologize, and I might become closer to others in the process.

How to apologize the right way

» A good apology is a genuine one. Say sorry and mean it.

» Acknowledge what you've done, perhaps offering an explanation for why it happened, and clearly state your sincere regret for the harm caused.

» There is no place in a good apology for counter-accusations or the words "but..." or "because you..."

» Support the words you use with eye contact, facial expressions, gestures and soft tones of voice.

How to accept an apology

» Look them in the eye and say...

"I forgive you."

If you feel you can, you can add the powerful words...

"Thank you for your apology."

EIGHT

GOALS & ACCOMPLISHMENTS

If you want to boost motivation, fine-tune focus or harness the power of shared purpose, then set some goals! There are many different applications of goal-setting, from creating big and challenging goals that stretch us as individuals to simply setting an intention for how you're going to spend the next half hour. Goals and intentions help kids get a handle on time, manage their expectations and create a sense of security, all of which boost health and well-being. This chapter isn't just about creating goals, it's also about pausing to reflect on achievements, big and small, because there is such zest to be mined there.

KEEP IT SIMPLE – FORMING INTENTIONS

When your children are little, the idea of setting goals with them might not initially resonate but, if you look at how you structure and navigate your day, you'll see it can be broken down into a set of mini goals. Children like certainty. They benefit from having structure to their day, providing a sense of familiarity and security in what's happening now and what's going to happen next, and clarity on what's expected of them. We can harness this by communicating with our kids a loose intention for periods of time, and giving warning of when the intention is changing to a different focus. This might seem rigid at first glance but, in reality, there is still plenty of fluidity and room for choice. Essentially this is bringing mindfulness and purpose to the flow of your day and having a dialogue with your family about it. Let me run you through our standard school day to demonstrate the flow of intentions. The phrase you'll hear repeated is "It's time to..."

» **Early morning.** It's time to wake, greet the day and each other. On tough mornings there are some rituals we use to boost energy and positivity, such as an extra-big cuddle in bed, a few yoga Mountain Breaths (see page 156) or thinking about one thing in our day that excites us.

» **Time to get ready for school** and the necessary activities (breakfast, toilet, teeth and dress). It's not time to play. It's not time to watch TV. If play is tempting, then we earmark the desired toys or games for after school, when it is time for play – it helps to know it will happen, just not right now. If we are *all* ready for school before we need to leave, then we can choose to play or watch TV. I've made this sound easy but I promise you, my house is just like yours...regularity and consistency do help.

goals & accomplishments

» Time to walk to school and we often engage in some kind of savouring activity to keep us focused on the journey – sometimes it is which birds can we see, how many cats or dogs can we count or looking for aeroplanes. If my kids are hesitant at the school gate we talk about some aspect of school they enjoy and set a positive intention together – it can be time to learn about something interesting or time with their friends.

» Afternoon reunion at school pick-up. It's time to connect and share what's happened in our day on the journey home. Then it's time for free play of their choosing and assisted homework.

» Dinner time. Five minutes prior to the end of play time I'll let my kids know that they have a few minutes left before transitioning to dinner time. I find that setting expectations in this way is much more effective than bellowing "Dinner time now" and the ensuing fight of getting them to the table. I don't like to be interrupted and told to drop things either, so some forewarning is less jarring and promotes greater cohesiveness and compliance. Let's be honest, there is often some cajoling required, but as my kids get older there's less resistance because they know the drill and why the next activity is important.

» Depending on timings there might be more play time or we move into time for bath and bed. This is often a tricky period for us because it's hard to put away the games and toys. I remind my kids that the fun is not over (which is a devastating thought for anyone!) – it's just this activity is done and it's time for something else. Bath time is enjoyable once they're in the tub and then we move into preparation for bed which is about soothing and connecting.

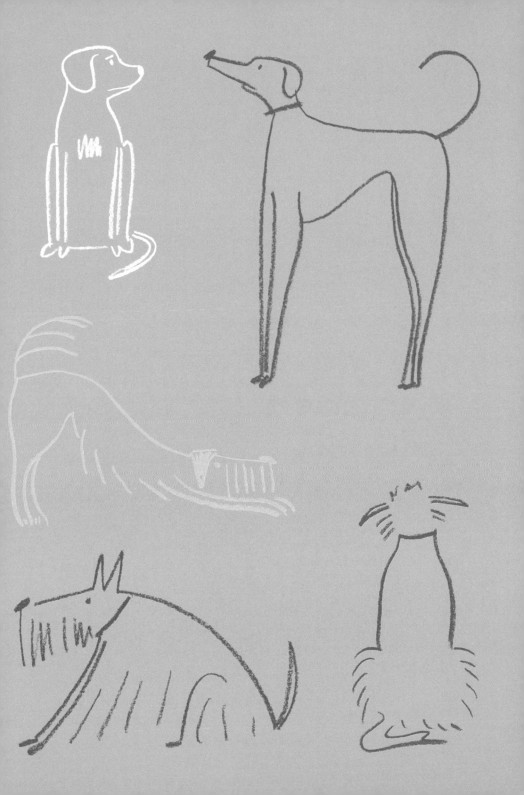

» **Bed time.** It's just time for rest and sleep. Sleep will come when it does and we use our "what to do when I can't sleep" toolkit on nights when this feels challenging (see page 72).

This approach helps us as parents to chunk down time. Rather than feeling you've got a whole day of "this" ahead, you've got this bit, followed by the next. Remind yourself your day can begin again in a breath. Don't wait for tomorrow for a fresh start. Setting an intention also makes it easier to more wholeheartedly devote your attention to work, parenting or other responsibilities. I find it helps me detach from the lure of my phone too.

To recap, by setting intentions for how we use our time and communicating these to our kids, we give them boundaries and a feeling of security. By saying "It is time for X" you are guiding your kids to what's expected of them and when they deviate we gently bring them back by saying "It's not time for that *now*", just like a mindfulness meditation, and if it's helpful, letting them know when it will be time for that desired activity. Connect them with what's to be enjoyed about this period, why you're doing what you're doing and get their buy-in. Distraction can see you through periods that aren't intrinsically interesting to your kids (necessary evils such as grocery shopping) and bribery will get you everywhere. Choice can be helpful too and sometimes as parents we have to turn to the illusion of choice. Offer a "choice" between carrots or peas, red socks or blue socks, or the opportunity to put their shoes on with help or on their own. You've got to do what you've got to do! While there will always be difficult periods, this is just the nature of family life. I hope this approach of making intentions will create a little more harmony to the flow of your day too.

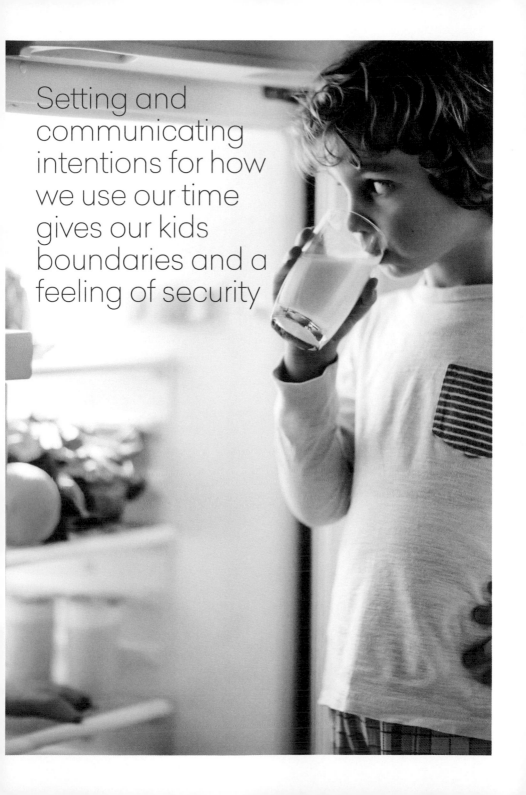

Setting and communicating intentions for how we use our time gives our kids boundaries and a feeling of security

GO FOR IT! SETTING GOALS

If you want to achieve anything, you are far more likely to do it if you create a goal for it. Goals refine your focus, give shape to your life and fire up your motivation. But not any goal will do. Research from Positive Psychology clearly shows that there are some principles that will help you craft a more life-giving goal. Sonja Lyubomirsky[16], an expert in happiness, summarizes these as follows:

1. The best goals are what you want for you, rather than what other people want for you.

2. To really galvanize you into action, make sure your goals tap into your values. Why do you want to achieve this goal – your "WHY" is your purpose and being clear on this gives you extra motivation and staying power.

5. Variables change all the time so make sure your goals are flexible and reasonable given the resources available.

4. Make sure your goals complement each other. It might not be possible to achieve all your goals at the one time and sometimes we need to prioritize or park some goals for later. Look for balance between your goals and those of your family members too.

3. It's better to frame your goals positively – what do you want to do more of rather than less of. For example, rather than say "I don't want to fight with my friend", reframe it as "I want to be kind and work on ways I can compromise with my friend".

goals & accomplishments

YOUR INDIVIDUAL GOALS & FAMILY GOALS

Defining and working toward your goals boosts not only your own personal happiness and well-being but sharing goals or the pursuit of goals with your family can also boost collective well-being. Sit down together and talk about what's important to each family member. Are there some loose intentions or goals you'd like to set as individuals? Just sharing your goals out loud can hold you accountable and increase your feeling of ownership of your aspirations. Making your intentions known will help people understand how to best support you and avoid unwittingly sabotaging your efforts. Consider how you can support each other in your individual goals. They may differ but you can still cheer each other on, building a feeling of connection and care.

Can you come together and create some collective goals – what's important to you as a family? Perhaps sifting through this book and the spokes of the Vitality Wheel might inspire you with some family goals. It can be anything from getting more movement into daily life, to exercising your mindfulness muscles, or simply having more fun together. Think about how you can each contribute toward this shared goal and talk about the actions you're each happy to commit to. Read the Strengths and Values chapter (from page 146) and think about how it could help you achieve your goals.

I've created a goal-setting plan to help you take action on your aspirations. You can fill this out for your individual goals or your shared family aspirations.

You are far more
likely to achieve
something if you
create a goal for it

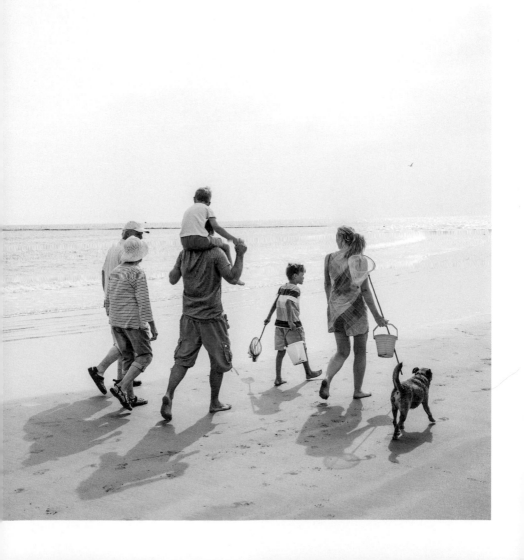

Harnessing the power of goal setting

My goal-setting plan

My goal
» I would like to achieve...

....

....

....

My WHY
» This is important to me because...
» When I achieve this I will feel...

....

....

....

My cheerleaders
» I will share my aspirations with...

....

....

....

Mini milestones

» What do I need to do to achieve my goal?

» Break it down into at least three mini action steps...
(Jot down some timeframes too if this is relevant)

....

....

....

Obstacles and strengths

» What might get in the way and what can I do to overcome them?

» Which of my strengths can I use to achieve my goal and cope
with setbacks?

....

....

....

Celebrate!

» How will I reward myself for each mini milestone and celebrate
my end goal?

....

....

....

Practice: Vision boarding

A great alternative to setting goals with words is using the power of imagery, creating a vision board. Children of any age can enjoy this approach and it can be a wonderful way of both sharing your dreams and building a feeling of shared hopes. A vision board is a collage of images that inspire you, representing what you'd like to achieve and what's important to you. It might include places you'd like to visit, activities you'd like to try or goals you've set for yourself and it affirms the values that lead the way. Creating a vision board can give you clarity on what's most important to you and having it in a prominent place will keep your goals fresh in your mind, fuelling your motivation. In creating a vision board you are priming your brain to achieve your aspirations so get as many of the senses involved as possible, imagining the action steps to get there and how it would feel for these dreams to become reality.

Making a vision board

First, gather your supplies. You'll need magazines, photos or printouts from the computer, pens, scissors, glue or tape and a large piece of paper or board to post your inspiration on. Share with your kids the intention of this project – to create a poster representing values and dreams for the future. You could inspire them with questions such as what kind of impact they'd like to have on the world, what they'd like to do when they grow up or what kind of super powers they would like to possess, as well as places they'd like to see or activities they'd like to do. Once they've had a chance to reflect, start sifting through the material you've gathered, clipping out images, words or phrases that resonate and arrange them on the board. Once the vision board is complete, sit down and talk through each image, asking what strength your children will call on or develop in working toward that vision. Break down into mini milestones what they can do to make their dreams a reality and highlight that we have to work to create these things for ourselves. Hang it up where it can easily be seen and give some gentle prompts about the agreed action steps.

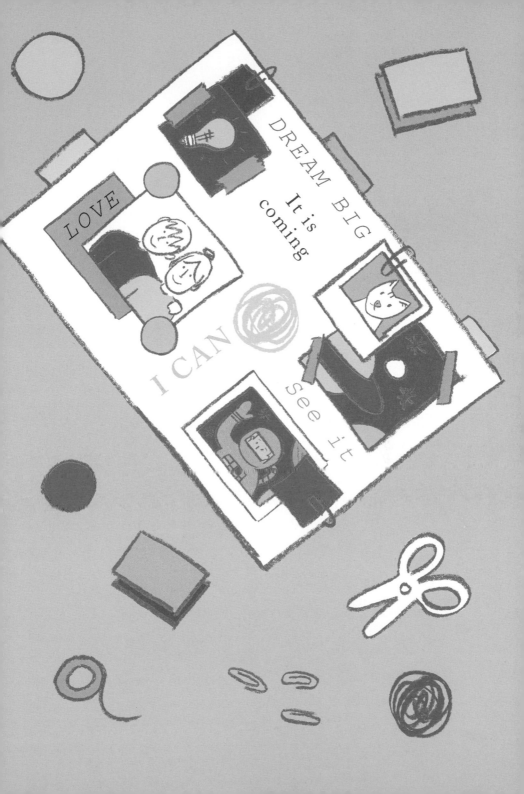

ACCOMPLISHMENTS

Once your child has achieved a task or goal, don't be in a hurry to zip onto the next thing. Encouraging them to notice their accomplishments lifts their spirits, gives them grit and boosts their self-esteem. Train their eyes to see what went well rather than what didn't pan out. We miss out on so much positivity by focusing on what's left undone. Encourage them to give themselves the pat on the back they deserve for their effort, even for the small things that are easy to brush off or overlook, like acquiring new everyday skills. If it is something of significance, reflect with your child on just how far they've come, the obstacles they've overcome, how they've grown along the way and then it needs to be celebrated! Parents, I appreciate the need for a "to do" list – I'd be lost without mine, but I think there's a place for the "what got done list" too. At the end of your day, run through all those tasks you knocked back and get good at using the mantra *"I appreciate me"*. For our children, it's easy to get lost in the mountain of homework and test preparation – make sure there is time to come up for air and celebrate good effort.

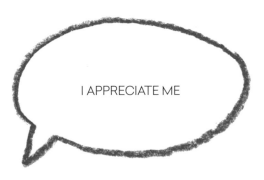

I APPRECIATE ME

Practices to harness the power of accomplishments

Reflect on your day and ask questions

"What went well and why?" This can be anything positive at all from "I listened well in English because I want to learn" or "I stood up for a friend at lunch because I value fairness". There is also no right or wrong to your "why" and this is an important part of the task because it boosts ownership and self-confidence.

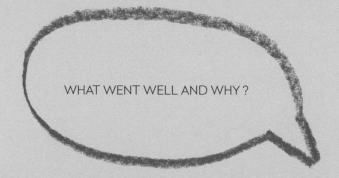

WHAT WENT WELL AND WHY ?

Some inspiration for your Self-Care Journal

Ponder the questions:

I can be proud of myself when I...

What is it about my family that makes me feel proud?

How am I proud of my friends?

What makes me feel proud of my team or school?

YOGA TO FIRE UP YOUR MOTIVATION AND REFLECT ON A JOB WELL DONE

PARTNERED STORK POSE

Purpose: to aspire and reach out for support along the way.

Facing your partner, hold hands and move as far away from each other as you can while keeping your hands clasped. Slowly raise one leg behind you and bring your spine parallel to the ground. Reach out, work toward your goal and feel the support of your partner as you navigate your way. Have a giggle too. Hold here for 5–10 breaths and then change legs. It's hard work but it's fun! You can also try this on your own. Don't worry if you wobble, it is all part of the journey.

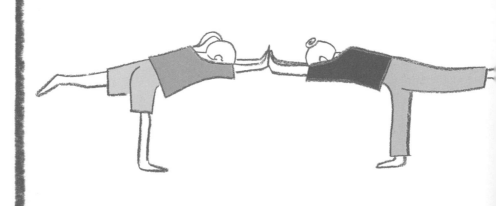

KNEELING LUNGE AND TWIST

Purpose: to be flexible and see things from different perspective.

Come down to all fours. Step your right foot forward toward your right hand. Place your hands on your front thigh and sink into the hip stretch, lengthening your out breath. See if you can just sit with the sensation without labelling it. Turn it into a Twist next by taking your left hand to the ground and raising your right arm skyward, looking up. Flexibility will help you become more malleable in your goal pursuit. Repeat on the other side. Enjoy a Ladybird pose (see page 68) or Downward Dog (see page 69) when you've done both sides.

LEGS UP THE WALL

Purpose: to stop and notice all you're achieving.

Lie down at the base of a wall and bring your legs up. Allow your legs to be completely relaxed and supported. Hang out here for at least five minutes, being with your breath, enjoying the absence of effort and basking in the glow of your efforts. Well done!

When I feel confused I will...

» Take a walk outside and blow out the cobwebs.

» Think about how I would like to feel. I'll look for a yoga pose in this book that might help me feel this way.

» Consider what I'd like to achieve in this situation. I can then break things down into little steps that might take me toward this.

» Think about my strengths and how they could help me right now.

» Focus on my values and what's important to me and see if that helps me think more clearly.

» Flip through the pages of my Self-Care Journal and see if something leaps out at me.

» Remind myself that it's ok to feel confused and I can talk to someone about how I'm feeling.

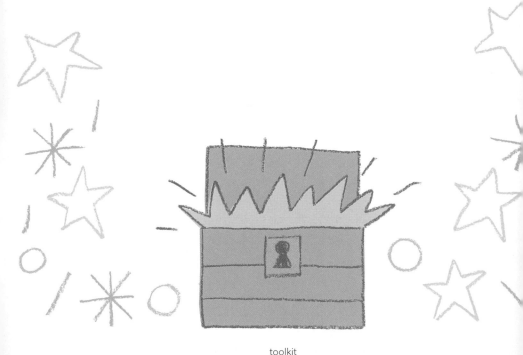

toolkit

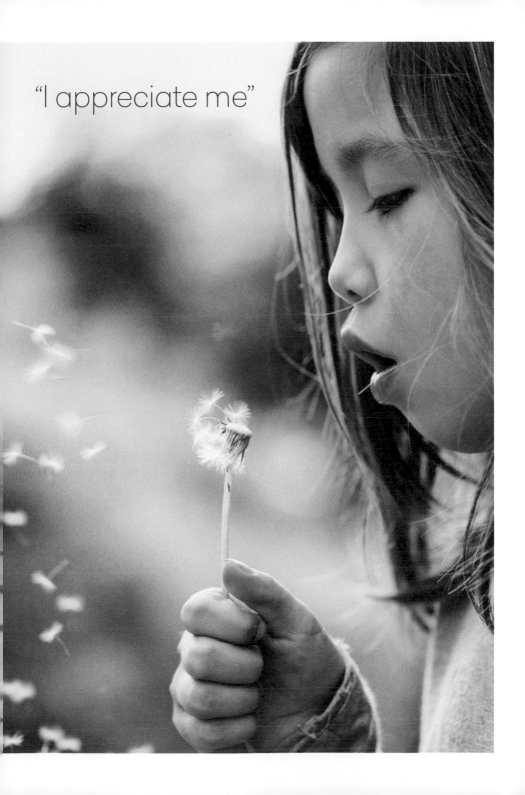

"I appreciate me"

WHAT NEXT?

· · · · · · · · ·

PAUSE & REFLECT

Don't do anything else, yet. Well done! Recognize the achievement it is to reach the end of this book, taking the time to empower yourself and your kids with nourishing habits. Bask in the glow of that accomplishment.

ACTION

Before you decide what you want to do, I want you to know that there have been times in my life when I've been so energetically bankrupt that it was all I could do to get my kids to school, fed and bathed. Vision boarding would have been nothing but a burden at that time in my life, so throw yourself a bone if you're in the midst of a tough time. Get the basics of self-care happening, nourishing you so you can keep giving and keep going. Save the other stuff for when energy returns – and it will. If your kids are at a low ebb, go gently. Prioritize the healing, soothing aspects of self-care for you and your family and I hope you will see the upward spiral of positivity swiftly set into motion. The yoga will help.

Some things in this book will resonate, some things may seem far-fetched, too saccharine sweet or just totally not up your alley. That's ok. What I do hope is that there might be one gem that significantly shifts your perspective and a handful of tools that will genuinely help you help your child. Our needs and interests are constantly changing, so the next time you flip through these pages something new might leap out at you.

Of the tools and tips that resonate, don't feel that you have to be doing all these things, all the time. I can safely say that all the strategies in this book I have learned the hard way, repeatedly, and I am still learning every day. A healthy dose of self-compassion will help us integrate these healthy habits ourselves and share them with our kids. Cut yourself some slack, dip into the book or turn to the Vitality Wheel and find something that will help you in the moment. Don't hesitate to reach out and seek support too. We all need it from time to time.

what next?

HOW TO CREATE CHANGE

One of the first places to start is annotating your Vitality Wheel with the ideas that resonate most for you and your family. Flip back through the chapters that interest you and jot down your favourite insights on the Wheel. Hang it up, check in with it regularly and use it to inspire you with a self-care practice when stress levels are rising. Even better, use it before then! Observe the collective mood of the household and proactively use the Vitality Wheel to determine the nourishment you need. With time, I hope you will notice that regularly engaging in self-care will make for greater collective patience and resilience, resulting in harmony and fewer, less intense eruptions.

Creating a Self-Care Journal for each family member will help you start to build your own personal toolkits. This will become a resource that your children can keep adding to and returning to for support. If your children can write, it is most effective when they note down their own lists of self-care activities and tools, forming a powerful primer statement. Knowing this toolkit is at fingertips' reach can greatly diminish anxiety – they will feel empowered by knowing what they'll do when faced with a particular challenge. Work with your children, using the suggestions in this book and your own ideas to create toolkits of what to do when challenges arise.

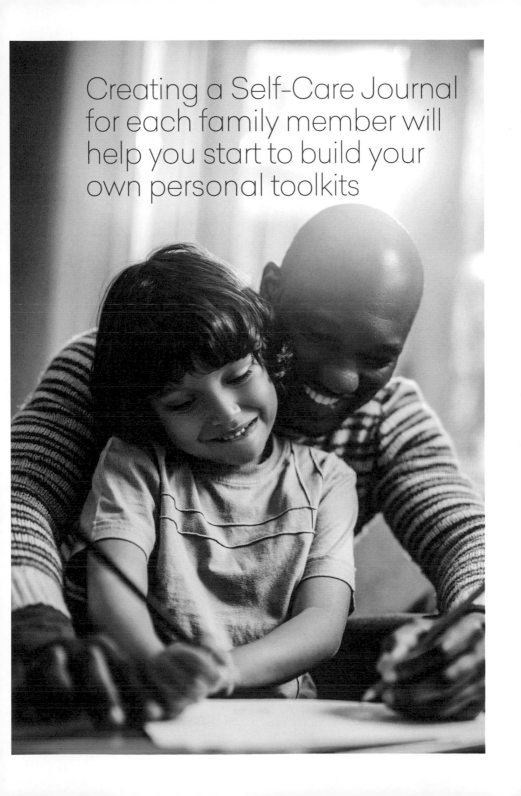

Creating a Self-Care Journal for each family member will help you start to build your own personal toolkits

Another idea is to loosely schedule in self-care. Do this lightheartedly. Let self-care be something to joyfully anticipate, not just another thing that needs doing. If you like, make appointments with yourself and with your kids and block out time in the calendar for fun and connection. This is important when life is very full or if you feel like you're missing out on time for family nurturing. Factor it in so it actually happens rather than waiting for that "good moment".

Are you and your family feeling ready for change? Which spokes of the Vitality Wheel call to you the most? Choose only two or three to work on at a time. You can revisit it once your first wave of change is integrated. Start small, work on one habit or tool at a time. The most effective way to make change is to break it down into small increments. If you'd like to clean up your eating, work on just one meal of the day rather than grand, sweeping change that's hard to implement and even harder to sustain. Use the Goals and Accomplishments chapter (page 160) to create your action plan. The best self-care is responsive and evolving, so keep your motivation fresh by returning to the book and asking what feels interesting to you now.

While this book is drawing to a close, our self-care journey together is just beginning. Thank you so much for spreading this self-care revolution with me. I hope you feel uplifted and nourished just reading about these concepts and that your self-care toolkit is now jampacked full of potent and accessible options. I hope you enjoy using it with your family and all the wonderful dividends it brings. I hope you all feel empowered to stand tall like a mountain.

Wishing you peace and ease.

We're in it together.

Suz xx

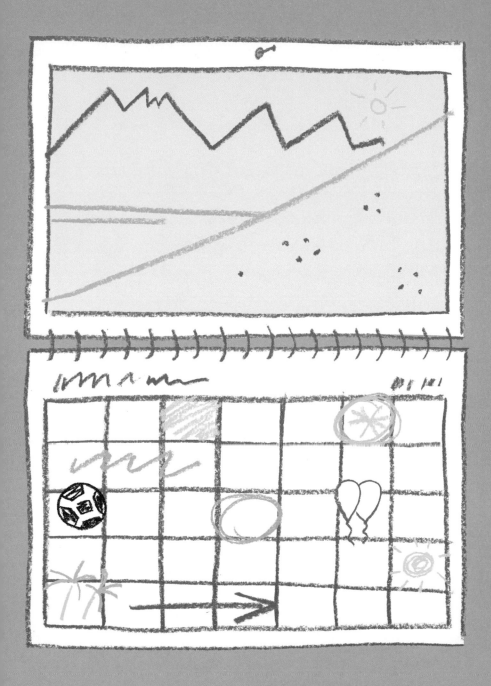

REFERENCES

1 Pond, R. S., Kashdan, T. B., DeWall, C. N., Savostyanova, A., Lambert, N. M., and Fincham, F. D., "Emotion differentiation moderates aggressive tendencies in angry people: A daily diary analysis", *Emotion*, 12, (2012) 326–337

2 https://www.linkedin.com/pulse/how-emotional-coach-7-tactics-help-your-child-tune-lea-waters-phd/

3 Dweck, Carol, Mindset: *The New Psychology of Success*, (New York: Random House, 2006)

4 https://news.harvard.edu/gazette/story/2011/01/eight-weeks-to-a-better-brain/

5 Harmon-Jones, E. and Peterson, C. K., "Supine body position reduces neural response to anger evocation", *Psychological Science*, 20(10), (2009), 1209–1210

6 Walsh, R., "Lifestyle and Mental Health", *American Psychologist*, Vol. 66, No. 7, (2011), 579 –592

7 Louv, R., *Last Child in the Woods: Saving Our Children from Nature-Deficit Disorder* (Chapel Hill: Algonquin Books, 2005)

8 Swamia, Viren, Barron, David, and Furnham, Adrian, "Exposure to natural environments, and photographs of natural environments, promotes more positive body image", *Journal of Body Image*, Vol. 24 (March 2018), 82–94

9 https://www.nutrition.org.uk/healthyliving/hydration/hydration-for-children.html

10 Carpenter, Siri, "That gut feeling", *Monitor on Psychology*, Vol. 43, no. 8, (September 2012)

11 Franzoi, Stephen L., "The body-as-object versus the body-as-process: Gender differences and gender considerations", *Sex Roles*, Vol. 33, Issue 5–6 (September 1995), 417–43

12 Abbott, B. D. and Barber, B. L., "Differences in functional and aesthetic body image between sedentary girls and girls involved in sports and physical activity: Does sport type make a difference?" *Psychology of Sport and Exercise*, 12 (3), (2011), 333–342.

13 https://youtu.be/xSe2h7fJgVg

14 https://www.tandfonline.com/eprint/eJz5eH7qiMmZCePXHWpE/full. Wallace, Sandi D. and Harwood, Jake, "Associations between shared musical engagement and parent–child relational quality: the mediating roles of interpersonal coordination and empathy", *Journal of Family Communication*, DOI: 10.1080/15267431.2018.1466783 (2018)

15 Waters, Lea, *The Strength Switch: How the New Science of Strength-based Parenting Helps Your Child and Your Teen Flourish*, (London: Scribe, 2017)

16 Lyubomirsky, S., *The How of Happiness*, (London: Piatkus, 2007)

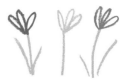

INDEX OF YOGA POSES

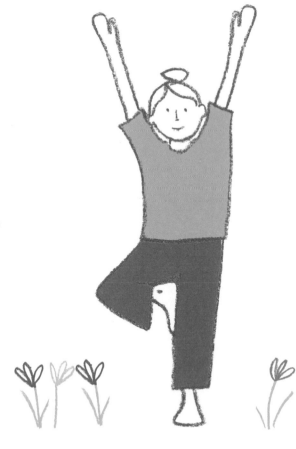

INDEX

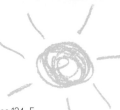

index

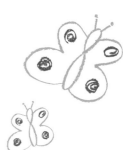

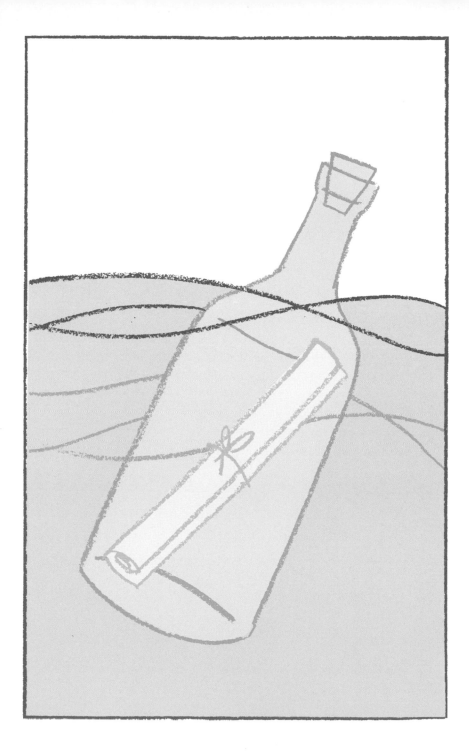

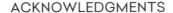

ACKNOWLEDGMENTS

Thank you to Mum, Dad, Michael and Robert, for giving me so early in a life such a secure base from which to explore the world. You instilled in me a great love of learning and appreciation of blessings that provide me with a tonic on a daily basis.

Thank you to my darling husband, Dave, for sharing this journey with me. Our achievements are always a team effort and I literally wouldn't be standing here without you. A huge debt of gratitude to you for your eternal love, support and encouragement to grow.

Thank you to Charlotte and Teddy – my greatest teachers. So many of the practices we created and fine-tuned together. A special thanks to Charlotte for helping me name the yoga poses. I hope these resources keep you well-nourished your whole life long.

To Donna, Charlotte, Danielle, Nikki, Clare, Emma and Laila – I am so grateful for your kindness and camaraderie. Every day is better for knowing we're in it together.

So much love to Liz Lark for sharing her yoga gems with me. They nourish me every day and that gift ripples out further from the yoga in the pages of this book. Thanks also to Ella Mclean for bringing my ideas to life with her beautiful illustrations.

To my agent, Jane Graham-Maw and Kate Adams, Pauline Bache and Megan Brown at Aster – a deep bow of gratitude for your belief, advocacy and support in getting my message out into the world.

Picture credits